Willem Einthoven (1860–1927)

Father of electrocardiography

Life and work, ancestors and contemporaries

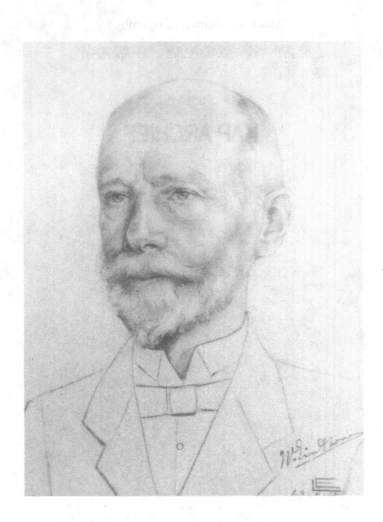

Portrait of Willem Einthoven (1860–1927) drawn by his grand-niece Lucie
Einthoven in April 1924. She was then only 13 years old. Later she made an artistic
and teaching career, and married fellow artist Moonen.
The original drawing was given by the Einthoven family to the Einthoven Foundation and is now on loan in the Einthoven collection of the Museum Boerhaave.

Willem Einthoven (1860–1927)

Father of electrocardiography

Life and work, ancestors and contemporaries

by

H. A. Snellen M.D.

Emeritus Professor of Cardiology,
University of Leiden, Leiden, The Netherlands

KLUWER ACADEMIC PUBLISHERS

DORDRECHT / BOSTON / LONDON

A C.I.P. Catalogue record for this book is available from the Library of Congress.

ISBN 0-7923-3274-1

Published by Kluwer Academic Publishers,
P.O. Box 17, 3300 AA Dordrecht, The Netherlands.

Kluwer Academic Publishers incorporates
the publishing programmes of
D. Reidel, Martinus Nijhoff, Dr W. Junk and MTP Press.

Sold and distributed in the U.S.A. and Canada
by Kluwer Academic Publishers,
101 Philip Drive, Norwell, MA 02061, U.S.A.

In all other countries, sold and distributed
by Kluwer Academic Publishers Group,
P.O. Box 322, 3300 AH Dordrecht, The Netherlands.

Printed on acid-free paper

Printed in the Netherlands

Contents

Contents

Introduction

Willem Einthoven (1860-1927); his life and work.

Introduction.

This is the first book on Einthoven in the English language; two earlier extensive reviews of his life and work were published in Dutch by his former co-workers Hoogerwerf and de Waart, in 1946 and 1957 respectively; the latter provides a brief summary in English; the former also wrote a succinct article on Einthoven in English.[74] Hoogerwerf's review[73] mentioned above was published as a chapter in "Helden der Wetenschap" i.e. "Heroes of Science," a book on Dutch Nobel Prize winners which has a somewhat romantic character corresponding with the title. On the other hand, de Waart's book[108] gives more scientific and technical details, and provides full reference to Einthoven's papers, his assistants and the doctoral theses written under Einthoven's guidance. On the whole therefore the latter is the best source of information and I have used it often and gratefully. At the same time it requires more effort to read; the other book may have had a wider reading public.

The main reason however for which I decided to write a book on Einthoven and was encouraged to do so by the Einthoven Foundation, is not the want of an English text, but the fact that more information has become available in the meantime. This consists of a) the Einthoven archive with a large and varied correspondence together with some personal notes, which Einthoven collected and arranged himself, and b) the privately printed history of the Einthoven family by Mr J.F.G. Einthoven[13], nephew of Willem Einthoven, who could profit from Mr P. Enthoven's investigations concerning the history of the Enthoven family from which the Einthoven branch descends (see chapter 1).

It is unfortunate that no former collaborator or friend of Willem Einthoven is left to write a new review of the latter's life and work. Some of his close acquaintances did publish their experiences on encountering Einthoven and visiting his laboratory; most of these papers are reviewed in chapter 6 of this book. They are chiefly written by Einthoven's colleagues and friends from abroad and published either in 1927 as an obituary or at some special date of commemoration such as 1960 (centenary of Einthoven's birth).

My own qualification for writing the present volume is at the same time limited and varied, i.e. linked with several isolated events that occurred long before I decided to start writing the present volume, some 4 years ago. For about 20 years I had then already studied various subjects from the history of cardiology after my retirement from the chair of clinical cardiology at Leiden University. In retrospect more important however, I am glad that I can say to have met several friends as well as former co-workers and relatives of Einthoven at much earlier occasions. Unfortunately I did not meet Einthoven himself although he was still alive and teaching at Leiden when I was a physical and later medical student in Utrecht, where Einthoven had studied himself.

My first contact with his laboratory, his equipment and his scientific heritage was in 1932 when I worked for a year with Einthoven's successor Rademaker in the Leiden physiological laboratory, prior to entering the medical department of Leiden University Hospital as an assistant who was supposed to concentrate on cardiology. The main interest of the laboratory was then focused on physiology of the central nervous system in particular reflexes concerning body positioning. Rademaker had been co-worker of Magnus at Utrecht, a famous pioneer in this field.

When I entered the laboratory, the large room with the different types of string galvanometers (to be described later) was still intact and I worked there with one of Einthoven's own string galvanometers coupled to an electronic amplifier. A combination which Einthoven himself had tried around 1920, but found unsatisfactory at that time. In 1932 it suited me well to study the electric responses from the inner ear which can be led off from the skull in response to the sound of a tuning fork.

Some of Einthoven's former co-workers still visited the laboratory once or twice a week during the morning coffee break, so I met them there (for instance Hoogerwerf who had established himself as a cardiologist at Leiden, but still was an unpaid university lecturer on physiology and the physicist Bergansius who had joined Einthoven's staff in 1911 and was now retired but overseeing the main clock, which had the nasty habit of getting a few seconds late in the course of a day). I met other former assistants in the following years outside the laboratory: two of them were general practitioners in the neighbourhood; Einthoven's biographer de Waart came back to Leiden from Indonesia in 1946 (see chapter 5), but already visited Holland several times in the 1930's.

Before that, in 1928 or 1929, I had visited Sir Thomas Lewis in his department at University College Hospital of London. Later, in the 1930's I met Wenckebach, Einthoven's younger companion of his student years, during some of his visits to his native country Holland where his sculptor son and one of his daughters lived as well as several pupils; also once in Germany where both of us were confronted for the first time with a Nazi official at a medical congress. The latter ridiculed some of the old leaders of the medical establishment from whom I remember Krehl. Wenckebach found this very funny, but he soon changed his opinion as I heard.

All this happened before the second world war. Other contemporaries of Einthoven especially those living in America, I met in 1946 when I had the good fortune to be included in a group of young cardiologists, sent by various European national societies of cardiology on the invitation of the Interamerican Congress of Cardiology. The latter convened at the wonderful new Institute of Cardiology (headed and planned by Chavez) at Mexico City. I rounded off this dazzling display of new cardiology (new at least to the recently liberated Europeans) by visiting the departments of some prominent cardiologists in the U.S.A. most of whom I had met in Mexico. Several of them knew Einthoven personally, or at least met him on his American tour in 1924. It was only much later that I realized how important these encounters with Einthoven's friends and contemporaries had been for my understanding of Einthoven's own papers and letters as well as those by others on him and to him respectively.

My attention was directed to Einthoven himself thanks to Paul White from Boston who in 1953 was preparing the Congress of the International Society of Cardiology for the following year at Washington. He asked me to talk about Einthoven in connection with the latter's paper of 50 years ago, that is of 1903 [31] in which the first electrocardiograms taken with the string galvanometer were published. I was ashamed that Leiden had to be reminded by the U.S.A. of its duty to cherish the memory of Einthoven, but happily it proved possible before the end of 1953 to organize a meeting at Leiden in which Nylin as (first) president of the European Society of Cardiology participated. Also Burger (of the Burger triangle) as well as de Waart and a few other former assistants of Einthoven who talked about their work with him and his string galvanometer. Several members of the Einthoven family were present.

After this meeting the University of Leiden instituted a two-yearly Einthoven Lecture which in 1979 led to the Einthoven Foundation for the study of the historical development of cardiology in relation to its current state. This happened after a very successful symposium on the history of such fairly recent topics as cardiac catheterization, angiocardiography and cardiac surgery with the participation of several respective pioneers who were still alive then (Forsmann who performed the first human heart catheterization on himself died just before the meeting, but his joint Nobel Prize winner Cournand was present; the latter attended many subsequent meetings at Leiden). From then on the Einthoven

Foundation organized a series of similar meetings in which usually an Einthoven Lecture was incorporated. Einthoven relatives from different generations continued to be present at these lectures.

To come back to the present volume: the first four chapters describe succinctly the four periods into which Einthoven's life and work can be divided in a natural way. Chapter 1 (1860-1885, but also including Einthoven's ancestry) deals with his youth at Semarang and Utrecht, in particular with his training at the Utrecht Medical School. Chapter 2 (1886-1900) reviews the first fifteen years at Leiden with their wide scientific orientation and gradual concentration on electrophysiology in particular of the heart, studied with Lippmann's capillary electrometer. Chapter 3 (1901-1916) relates the construction of the string galvanometer and its applications, especially to the development of electrocardiography. Chapter 4 (1917-1927) is concerned with the final perfecting of the string galvanometer, its limitations and various applications, in particular the reception of radiotelegraphic signals from the Dutch East Indies. The by then general recognition of Einthoven's work will also be mentioned together with his lecture tour in the United States and the posthumous publication of his review of electrocardiography.

In accordance with the subtitle of this book Einthoven's relation with well acquainted contemporaries is examined in chapters 5 and 6; they contain a selection of Einthoven's correspondence with colleagues and friends, co-workers and relatives as well as some papers by them on Einthoven. The two chapters are subdivided into sections comprising information about the respective correspondents and the letters exchanged with them. Chapter 5 contains correspondence in Dutch, which in practice means the early correspondence. The letters in German and English (chapter 6) were chiefly written after the publication of the string galvanometer. However, Waller was an exception as an early English correspondent, while some Dutch correspondents prolonged their written contact for several years after the turn of the century. The papers bearing on Einthoven and his work which I selected for discussion and quotation were chiefly published by correspondents from other countries and therefore reviewed in chapter 6.

Chapter 7 discusses additional (and in general more recent) evaluations of Einthoven and his work, together with a brief review of some correspondence with firms about manufacturing the string galvanometer commercially, notably Edelmann. It will be shown in chapter 7 that - as could be expected - knowledge of Einthoven and his work diminished in course of time; but it also became distorted: by failing memory, unchecked quoting or incomplete and superficial reading. Concluding remarks terminate this book.

In order to show how far the ignorance about Einthoven had progressed, Ershler in 1988 [64] reported that he asked many doctors and medical students what they knew of Einthoven and his work. The best answer was a question: "Wasn't he someone who had something to do with a triangle?"; see chapter 3 and Einthoven's paper on the equilateral triangle[46]. Ershler's conclusion that people should be told anew was correct of course, but his own attempt to do so was chiefly based on information from his former chief George Fahr with addition of a few quotations from A.V.Hill (both authors are discussed in chapter 6). Unfortunately several "facts" reported by Fahr are unreliable (in contrast to Fahr's personal observations) as chapter 6 will show.

At any rate, it is important that publications on Einthoven can now be checked on the basis of his own archive. It has served Burnett already in preparing his paper[9] and hopefully also will benefit others, especially when the most interesting parts will have been made more easily available. It is a rich archive mostly consisting of correspondence together with personal notes, drafts for publications or speeches, but also material received by Einthoven in the form of papers, reports, prospectuses etc.

The correspondence itself is very extensive and concerns a great number of persons and institutes, varying from isolated letters (often demanding permission to see the string galvanometer or inquiring where it could be bought) to long continued exchange of letters. Of the latter type of correspondence there are three which cover twenty years or more; in two cases (Lewis and Samojloff) with gaps of a few years in the middle due to World War I and its aftermath; in the third (Waller) with many substantial gaps but spread out over more than thirty years.

Both the correspondence with Thomas Lewis of London, and with Alexander Samojloff of Kasan (Russia) start by expressing their wish to visit Einthoven's laboratory and to see the string galvanometer (in 1908 and in 1904 respectively); in both cases also with the intention to obtain a string galvanometer for their own research, which makes them early pioneers of electrocardiography. Lewis, a clinician besides a brilliant experimentist, is the best known of the two; his correspondence also is scientifically the most interesting. The correspondence with Lewis was fully published in 1983. [102]

Samojloff was a physiologist with predominant interest in heart action currents like Einthoven himself; he ranks among the first who published on electrocardiography (including a small book: Elektrokardiogramme, 1909 [96]). His correspondence however is mostly of a personal character; in particular after the Russian revolution when he repeatedly asked for help which Einthoven delivered readily in spite of his own heavy work load. Both collections of letters will be discussed in chapter 6.

The third long lasting correspondence (also reviewed in chapter 6) is that with A.D. Waller from London. Although it stretches from 1890 to 1921 it is not very extensive, because of large gaps between the letters. Interesting are the close similarity in some respects and large discrepancies in other ways between Waller's and Einthoven's work (and also between their respective personalities and life-style). Moreover and most essential, Waller's demonstration of the human heart's action current opened the door to the central theme of Einthoven's career.

What makes these and many other parts of the correspondence especially valuable as documentation, in particular concerning the period prior to 1920, i.e. before Einthoven had a secretary with a typewriter who made copies, is that Einthoven himself already well before 1900 copied his own letters or at least wrote the gist of them on the paper of the letters he was answering.

It is likely that Einthoven's copies were made by inserting a wet piece of paper under the freshly written letter so as to make the ink of the letter penetrate into the underlying paper, when a roller was applied to the letter itself. The results of the first 1-2 years (around 1895) of this procedure are very difficult to read because of blotting; moreover,the paper of these copies is now crumbling, making photographic recording an urgent matter. The procedure was probably the same as used in London at that time as I was told by Dr Arthur Hollman, but Lewis never kept copies of his own letters; nor is his collection of letters from Einthoven complete (the Lewis archive is now at the Wellcome Institute, London).

Some parts of Einthoven's correspondence are important in revealing Einthoven's intentions, his opinions (in particular about himself) and his working methods. This holds also for the understanding of Einthoven's publications, which although clearly and simply formulated, sometimes have been misunderstood; partly perhaps because of insufficient and careless reading. Moreover it is true, that Einthoven himself did not mention some facts or conclusions which he supposed to be generally known or self-evident. In chapter 6 it will be set forth that Wilson later felt obliged to assist readers by writing a few papers explaining Einthoven's intentions.

Perhaps I should add here that Einthoven used to write most of his papers in several languages, usually first in Dutch then in French and/or German or (less frequently) in English (see also chapter 5, section 2). This was not uncommon in Einthoven's time; his teacher Donders did the same, wanting to reach a widely varied reading public. Lewis however in 1921 wrote to Einthoven that he never published the same matter twice; his choice of a subject for a lecture at Leiden therefore was difficult to make, if the lecture had to be published afterwards.

The present volume could only be finished thanks to the kindness and support I received from the staff of the Museum Boerhaave, the interest and generosity of the Einthoven Foundation and the information from various members of the Einthoven family, several of whom are now already part of a cherished memory. Essential and highly appreciated was the secretarial help of Mrs Tetteroo from the Einthoven Foundation and her predecessors, but also often of my wife.

I am much indebted to the friends and colleagues who assisted me by procuring documents and other information or by reading part of the work while it was in progress (e.g. Prof. Tammeling , one of Einthoven's later successors). In the final stage much needed and helpful support was given by Prof. Janse at Amsterdam and my own two successors Professors Arntzenius and Bruschke and the latter's secretarial staff.

Acknowledgement.
I am grateful to the late Mrs Einthoven-Zeeman and the late Miss M. Wenckebach, the Wellcome Institute at London, Boerhaave Museum at Leiden, Archives of the city of Leiden, Department of Physiology and Academic Hospital of the University of Leiden and the Einthoven Foundation for their courtesy in supplying illustrations.

Chapter one (1860-1885).

Willem Einthoven's ancestors. Early childhood at Semarang; school-days and medical training at Utrecht.

Around the middle of the 18th century the Jewish merchant David Joseph left the Palatinate on the banks of the river Rhine, after its ruler in 1744 had issued a decree limiting the number of Jews in his state. David Joseph settled in Eindhoven, then a small town, in Holland. When he subsequently moved to the Hague, he occasionally called himself Enthoven; presumably using the name of the town where he came from, as a means of identification. Later his eldest son Juda David moved to neighbouring Delft. In 1806 Napoleon occupied Holland and made it a kingdom for his brother Louis Napoleon, but in 1810 he annexed it to France as a province. The Code Napoléon required all inhabitants to choose and officially adopt a last name for themselves, their wives and their children. Juda David had died by that time but among those who had to obey the rule, was his brother Israel David with his wife, who chose the name of Enthoven. From Juda David's two sons, one simplified his name to Hoven and the other - who was to become Willem Einthoven's grandfather - made a slight change from Salomon Juda Enthoven to Salomon Jurdan Einthoven after he went to England. There he was trained in surgery and became assistant military surgeon of the King's German Legion. The latter was mainly recruited from Hannover, where the King himself came from. The purpose of the legion was to assist in the fight against Napoleon. It participated in the resistance to Napoleon's invasion of Italy and especially Spain; later it joined in the battle of Waterloo. Thereafter the legion was disbanded and Salomon Jurdan Einthoven went back to Holland. Not to the Hague or Delft where most of his relatives lived but to Groningen, far away in the north of the country. There he started a surgical practice after having passed the required examination. He became a member of the Dutch Reformed Church and married the eldest daughter of the professor of physics and astronomy at the University of Groningen, called Baart de la Faille. Salomon Jurdan Einthoven stayed at Groningen until his death in 1850. His wife, who bore him 5 children (among them Jacob, Willem Einthoven's father), died in 1828 from puerperal fever after ten years of marriage[a]. Salomon Jurdan remarried to her younger sister after having obtained the legally needed permission.

Son Jacob studied medicine at Groningen with a grant from the government which required a contract to serve for 10 years in the army. He chose to pass this period in the Dutch East Indies (now Indonesia). A 13 years younger half-brother later followed his example but took medical military service as a career and was trained at the army's medical school at Utrecht. Together they established the tradition of a tropical career in the Einthoven family which resulted in the continued presence of some members of the family in the East Indies during the next 100 years or so. Jacob left Holland for Batavia (now Djakarta) in 1846 on board of a sailing vessel for a voyage around the Cape of Good Hope; such a journey took almost 4 months. After the construction of steamships and the opening of the Suez canal a regular service was established between Holland and the Dutch East Indies in the 1870's. The time needed for the journey was then reduced to less than four weeks.

Jacob Einthoven performed his military service in various parts of the Dutch East Indies; his last position before the contract expired was at the Military Hospital of Semarang, an important harbour on the island Java. After leaving the army Jacob became second town physician of Semarang.

Like many of his contemporaries Jacob Einthoven had arrived in the tropics as a bachelor and started living with his native housekeeper. She bore him 4 children whom he recognized and kept at his home, when she died (or perhaps left) after her last confinement. Subsequently he married a Dutch girl, whose father was tax director at Semarang. Mrs Einthoven thus started her marriage with four stepchildren; in the course of the following 10 years she had six of her own. The last one - a girl - was born after Jacob's early death from a stroke in 1866; Willem Einthoven was then 6 years old. Jacob's half-brother who followed the former's footsteps, had arrived at Semarang in 1859 and was trained in the same Military Hospital where Jacob had been stationed. Later the younger two of Jacob's sons both chose a career of civil service in the Dutch East Indies and Willem Einthoven himself, the oldest son, initially planned a medical career there.

The educational facilities in the tropics were limited and on a higher level non-existent at the time. It was the custom of Dutch residents to return to

---

[a] When Jacob wrote his (Latin) doctoral thesis of medicine in 1846, its title was "De peritonitide puerperali".

Holland at the end of their career, but to send their children (at least the sons) back as soon as high school and further training were required. Mrs Einthoven's stepson had already left for that purpose, the oldest of his three sisters had married and the second also had left home, when Jacob's widow with the rest of the children and a niece in 1870 went back to live at Utrecht. The party also included Mrs Einthoven's bachelor brother, who continued to stay with her after arriving in Holland.

A few years later Willem and subsequently his younger brother went to a recently introduced type of high school which provided a shorter preparation for academic studies by omitting Latin and Greek while adding some more science (and later economics). It took 50 years however, before the graduates who had entered university from that type of school were given the right to submit a formal doctor's thesis; the requirement of a Latin text for such a thesis had already been abolished long before that. When Willem became aware of that obstacle, he studied classical languages and took a supplementary examination after finishing high school. This exercise earned him a lifelong interest in Latin literature, from which he could recite many passages, as Fahr testified[67].

His medical studies were also carried out at Utrecht, where eminent scientists were able to captivate his interest, although not always his approval. In fact, on the two occasions that Einthoven distinguished himself as a student, his main achievement consisted in reaching conclusions which were based on his own observations and calculations but differed from those of his teachers. For the first time this occurred after an accident during gymnastics, whereby he broke his wrist. (Einthoven was an all-round sportsman in those days; he was also one of the founders and active members of the students' rowing club). In order to regain a good function of his hand he practised fencing. He vied with his brother, who was training at Delft for civil service in the Dutch East Indies, for the first prize in the fencing competition of Dutch students and won. At the same time his temporary handicap drew his attention to pronation and supination of the elbow, which he studied geometrically and in observations on himself; he arrived at conclusions on the rôle of the shoulder joint in this connection, which were opposed to the teaching of his professor in anatomy[14]. The latter showed appreciation however and presented Einthoven's paper to the Dutch Royal Academy of Sciences.

Something similar happened when Einthoven challenged the views of Donders on the cause of the seeming difference in depth of red and blue letters attached to a black screen; an optical illusion which Donders had perceived in a hotelroom at Leipzig, when he visited Ludwig in his famous laboratory. Donders was both a well known physiologist and a pioneer of ophthalmology. He founded at Utrecht the first Dutch hospital for diseases of the eye. In 1883 his clinical responsibilities had been turned over to his assistant Snellen (of the Snellen Tables, my grandfather), who was given the recently founded chair of ophthalmology while Donders concentrated on physiology in a new and well equipped laboratory. Einthoven, planning to go to the Dutch East Indies like his father and to introduce there the speciality of ophthalmology, had started to assist Snellen at the Eye Hospital where Donders still was director. Einthoven's contact with Donders was intensified in this way.

The latter used to demonstrate in his lectures the optical illusion mentioned above and ascribed the impression of different depth of equidistant red and blue letters to different accommodation for red and blue light. It appeared however that some persons did not share this illusion (or not to the same degree) and Einthoven was one of them. Donders suggested to Einthoven the study of this phenomenon.

Einthoven carried out a series of observations in 32 normal volunteers of different age and sex (among them Donders and Snellen with their wives) while covering part of their pupil. Together with mathematical constructions these experiments showed that asymmetrical position of the pupil with respect to the eye was essential for a stereoscopic effect, which disappeared if one eye was closed. Hence the title of "Stereoscopy through difference in colour" of Einthoven's doctoral thesis[15,16] which was received "cum laude" although it contained only 32 pages.

These events indicated already a remarkable aspect of Einthoven's mind, i.e. his ability to recognize the essential character of a problem which he happened to meet, as well as his persistent curiosity which drove him to go to the bottom of the problem as far as possible. His fellow students were impressed, as Wenckebach, a younger contemporary of Einthoven at Utrecht - later himself professor of medicine at Groningen, Strassbourg and Vienna - remembered. In Einthoven's obituary[117] Wenckebach wrote: "Man ahnte schon den kommenden Mann". (One could already imagine the coming man). Einthoven's preference for physical and mathematical methods was going to reveal itself many times again after this. Perhaps inheritance played a rôle, as both his grandmother's father and grandfather were physicists.

In the same year 1885 in which Einthoven obtained his doctoral degree, the chair of physiology at Leiden became vacant. After refusal by a previous

chief assistant of that laboratory (as Einthoven himself later revealed in the former's obituary), Einthoven was offered this position. Very likely his nomination
at such a young age was at least partly due to the influence of Donders whose
opinion carried much weight. As mentioned before, Einthoven intended to go to
the Dutch East Indies like his father, and had accepted a study grant from the
government. These initial plans now caused some difficulty because the pro-
fessorship at Leiden implied the gradual repayment of his study grant of fl. 6.000
from a yearly salary as young professor of fl. 4.000 (de Waart[108]). Einthoven
accepted nevertheless; he finished his studies by taking his medical licence at
Amsterdam and assumed his duties at Leiden early in 1886, still aged 25. He was
going to stay there for the rest of his life.

Two months after his inaugural address (on Müller's doctrine of specific
energies, i.e. specific abilities of the sense organs) Einthoven married his cousin
Louise de Vogel. She was to survive her husband for 10 years. One son and three
daughters were born from this marriage. The son studied electric engineering and
while still a student, collaborated with his father, particularly in a highly ambi-
tious project of radiotelegraphy which will be discussed in Chapter 4.

Chapter two (1886-1900).

Scientific orientation and self-study at Leiden. Gradual concentration on electrophysiology in particular of the heart, using Lippmann's capillary electrometer.

As in other universities, physiology at Leiden was an offspring of anatomy; it still comprised another speciality emerging from anatomy, i.e. histology. Although Einthoven never performed specific histological research, he used to give the lectures on histology himself and acquired knowledge of microscopical structure which later proved very useful (e.g. for understanding the importance of the conducting system as soon as it was discovered and also for identification of the cellular origin of cardiac action potentials, to be discussed later). In 1906 a reader of histology was appointed: Dr Boeke, who took over the lectures in histology, until he was called to Utrecht as professor in histology. After Einthoven's arrival two co-workers of his predecessor continued their research; one of them a histologist, the other a biochemist.

A chair for medical biochemistry was instituted after Einthoven's death. From a letter to his friend and brother-in-law Julius dated Nov. 26, 1896 it is clear that Einthoven had mixed feelings about promoting the establishment of a chair in biochemistry at the same time as in histology. He foresaw that its department would have to be lodged in the physiological laboratory (histology was put up in the anatomical laboratory) and therefore would imply loss of space and freedom. Especially space was an important problem, which Einthoven around 1890 had been able to solve by creating a large room through glass-roofing of the laboratory's inner yard. It was in this room that Einthoven housed his capillary electrometers and later his successive types of string galvanometer. In 1896 Einthoven introduced the first volume in his own series of collected publications (as a sequel to that of his predecessor) by giving some information about the laboratory (fig.1), mentioning the construction mentioned above, which provided excellent light and the opportunity to erect large stone pillars in order to protect sensitive instruments against extraneus oscillations; moreover the building of a shed and a new inner yard.
At the same time he stressed the need of an extensive electrical installation for which an annex was built after or around 1900 (fig.2).

Initially Einthoven's personal research concerned the two fields which he had become familiar with in Donders' laboratory, i.e. vision and respiration.

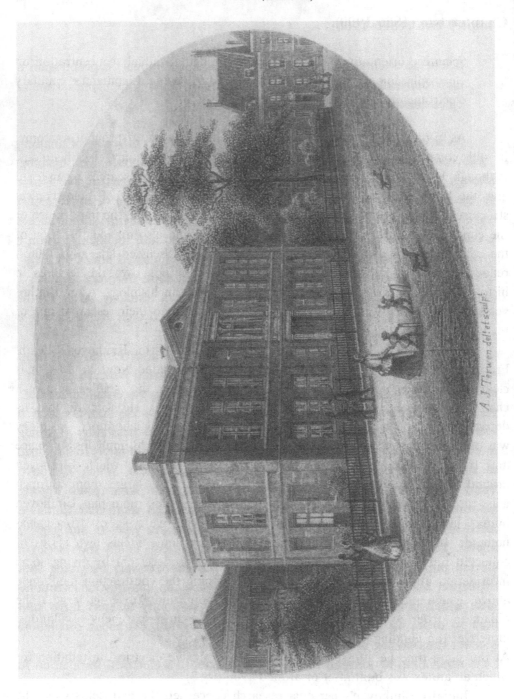

The latter subject had also been one of the main topics of previous work in the Leiden laboratory. His optical studies partly continued the investigation of optical illusions as embodied in his thesis, especially after A.D. Waller informed him that he had obtained the illusion of difference in depth of two colours with one eye shut, after the pupil of the other eye was made eccentric. Einthoven found that the phenomenon could indeed be produced with one eye looking at two differently coloured sheets, if they partly covered each other so as to produce a shadow when viewed under a slanting light. The difference in colour increased the shadow and made it seem that there was a difference in depth, depending on the direction of the light. The decisive factor in this case proved to be that the observer supposes the light to come from the usual (frontal) direction instead from the side[20]. Subsequently optical illusions were going to attract Einthoven's attention at several occasions. One of them concerned a tiled wall alongside the staircase in the pathological laboratory at Leiden. (This staircase later became part of the Boerhaave Museum until the latter's move to the renovated Cecilia hospital, where Boerhaave used to teach at the bedside). These tiles consisted of a neat arrangement of alternating greater and smaller squares in white or in black with white border on a black background which produced the impression of a chaotic disarray.

In the "Festschrift" for Donders on the latter's 70th birthday which marked his retirement (1888 followed by his death within a year), Einthoven studied the mechanism of maintenance of the normal negative (i.e. below atmospheric) intrapleural pressure discovered by Donders himself, and its change in pneumothorax. Einthoven did so by constructing a curve from measurements of the intrapleural pressure after injection and withdrawal of known quantities of air and extrapolating therefrom. At the same time he measured the different rates of production and absorption of the gases composing the air contained in the interpleural space[17]. Subsequently he went to the laboratory of marine biology at Naples to study the gases in the swimming bladder of fishes (although his medical faculty refused to support his application for a grant relating to this project, according to de Waart[108]).

In 1892 Einthoven published his most important respiratory research,

---

Figure 1 (opposite page) . *Front of the physiological laboratory Leiden (25 years or so before the arrival of Einthoven). Initially it comprised anatomy and physiology.*

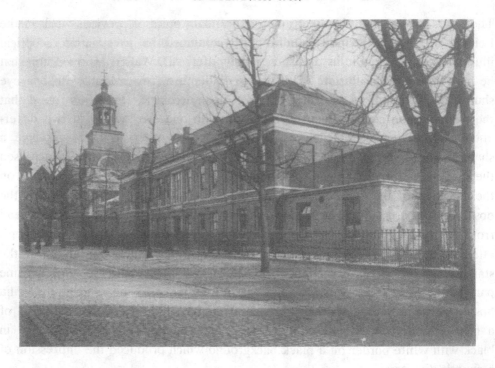

Figure 2. *Front of the physiological laboratory Leiden (around 1920) with added annex for electrical installation at the right.*

which concerned the experimental proof of bronchial constriction by vagal stimulation.

Bronchial spasm was already accepted as cause of bronchial asthma (then called asthma nervosum) by most clinicians, particularly after the publication by Biermer in 1870 [6], but refuted by most physiologists because it had not been proven experimentally or was considered negligible.

In his investigation Einthoven periodically and automatically injected into the lungs of some curarized dogs and/or with opened chest a constant quantity of air while measuring the intratracheal pressure during in- and expiration. The intratracheal pressure could be used in this way as an indication of bronchial constriction. To complete his experimental investigation Einthoven was given the opportunity to observe some patients during an asthmatic attack and interviewing them afterwards.

The third essential element in this research was a theoretical review of changes during respiration of the forces which respectively dilate or narrow the (smaller) airways, dependent on the phase of respiration (in- or expiration) and its intensity (forceful or light). This theoretical part was illustrated and summarized by a schematic graph wherein a family of curves was drawn that showed the various types of respiration and their effects on the lumen of the airways.

In respiratory standstill and open glottis the pressure is the same in all parts of the airways and is equal to atmospheric pressure. During respiration, the alveolar pressure is negative i.e. below atmospheric like the interpleural pressure, which was first measured by Donders (see above). On inspiration pressures fall, particularity in the dilating smaller and somewhat larger bronchi according to the depth of inspiration. On expiration the bronchial lumen is more or less compressed and the pressure therein will be higher and positive (above atmospheric) as soon as the expiration becomes forceful.

In an asthmatic attack the bronchi are narrowed by mascular constriction. Moreover the lungs become hyperinflated (experimentally confirmed by vagal stimulation) which tends to compress the bronchi still more. The effect of electrical stimulation of the vagus on bronchial constriction is short-lived but as Einthoven pointed out, the asthmatic attack is likely to cause accumulation of CO_2 in the blood, thereby stimulating the vagal centre in the brain. In this way a vicious circle way can arise which prolongs bronchial constriction and the asthmatic attack.

In addition Einthoven made the interesting statement that such a vicious circle can also occur in other states of respiratory or circulatory deficiency. Clinical relevance was suggested, although the term cardiac asthma was not used and advice on diagnosis or treatment (e.g. by atropin) was explicitly refrained from.

The conclusion was made by Einthoven however from the experimental evidence (and his limited clinical observations) that in an asthmatic attack inspiration will have to be maximal, while expiration must be quiet and slow because forceful expiration will narrow the bronchi. This view was opposed to the prevailing opinion of clinicians who regarded expiratory distress as the main aspect of dyspnea in an asthmatic attack. Einthoven realized that: "Es dürfte einigermaassen kühn erscheinen dass der Theoretiker am Schreibtisch den Kliniker, wo es dessen Wahrnehmungen am Krankenbette betrifft, verbessern zu können glaubt" (It may appear somewhat bold that the theorist at his writing-table thinks that he can correct the findings of the clinician at the bedside).

The first reactions came sooner, from another side and more aggressively than Einthoven must have anticipated (from von Basch and Grossmann both from Vienna; again in Pflüger's Archiv of the same year 1892). Apparently these physiologists felt that their work was misrepresented and underestimated by Einthoven; they mounted a fierce and rather personal counter attack, especially Grossmann. In retrospect Einthoven's criticism of the earlier physiological literature on this subject appears sound and objective, although perhaps a little too explicit and unvarnished for a young unknown professor; but the authors mentioned above were indignant. Einthoven did not respond to this or other criticism; a year later when speaking to a Dutch medical audience, Einthoven[22] while maintaining his conclusions, called the opposition chiefly based on misunderstanding and announced his plans to answer it, using new experiments which were already being prepared (but never published and probably left unfinished). In later years his paper got little mention until it was rediscovered by two Dutch authors: Dekker in his thesis of 1958[11,12] who saw it as an important contribution to the understanding of asthma and bronchial (patho)physiology, later followed up by Tammeling[105] in his paper at the Einthoven symposium of 1977, which commemorated the latter's death in 1927.

Perhaps this early experience in 1892 mentioned above was (partly) responsible for some later statements by Einthoven as for instance in his Dutch obituary of Marey[32] in 1904 where he praised Marey as exceptional by never meeting with personal attacks in literature or discussions nor making any such attacks himself. There also may be a relation with Einthoven's statement 20 years later as reported by Wiggers (see chapter 6, section 7), i.e. that investigators perhaps should spend more energy on harmonizing divergent results than on defending earlier conclusions by new experiments.

Almost at the same time (1891) Einthoven's brother-in-law Willem de Vogel whom Einthoven had supported during his medical studies according to de Waart[108], came to work in the physiological laboratory in order to prepare his doctoral thesis. From the possible subjects which Einthoven proposed to him, de Vogel chose that of cardiac electrical activity. This topic was a new one as far as the examination of human subjects was concerned.

A.D. Waller[110] was the first to demonstrate the cardiac currents in man and intact animals (at a meeting of the Physiological Society at London in 1887). Waller later said that Einthoven was present there, but confirmation of this statement has not been found either at London (Sykes[103]) or at Leiden. In 1895

Einthoven himself[24] only quoted the published account of Waller's demonstration (1887 [110]) and the latter's subsequent extensive paper of 1889 [111]. It is certain however, that Einthoven saw Waller's demonstration at the first international physiological congress (Bâle 1889), because he wrote a report of that congress, in particular of Waller's contribution, for the main Dutch medical journal (Nederlands Tijdschrift voor Geneeskunde)[18]. After Waller, Bayliss and Starling published in 1892 human electrocardiograms (their own) in an appendix to their paper on experimental research in cardiac electrophysiology[5]. In 1891 de Vogel started to study electrical action currents in the exposed heart of frogs, rabbits and a dog, with and without the application of drugs (digitalin, muscarin, atropin). Subsequently he examined 2 human hearts, his own and that of the chief technician in a lead from the two hands. In the meantime Einthoven occupied himself with the analysis and improvement of the apparatus used by Waller, i.e. Lippmann's capillary electrometer [a] and its photographic registration, introduced by Marey. Although de Vogel in his thesis of 1893[107] mentions that the glass capillary of his electrometer was made according to the requirements calculated by Einthoven, the human tracings in de Vogel's thesis still show small deflections; much smaller than those Einthoven himself obtained slightly later. Both however surpassed Waller's tracings considerably in size and definition. Moreover Einthoven's subsequent tracings displayed 4 peaks (ABCD) instead of the 2 found by Waller, de Vogel and initially also Einthoven himself. The remarks of Wiggers[119] on the different quality of Waller's and Einthoven's electrocardiograms will be quoted in chapter 6, section 7.

Because I received some inquiries about the introduction of the term electrocardiogram and its orthography, I feel that I should add the pertinent information. The term electrocardiogram was coined by Einthoven who used it for the first time in a paper at the general meeting of the Dutch medical association of 1893[21], in which he spoke of two new clinical methods (i.e. E.C.G. and phonocardiogram). The word electrocardiogram was spelt with two C's; the same happened in subsequent papers in English, French (électrocardiogramme) and German (Electrocardiogramm). In 1900 the latter was changed into Elektrokardiogramm with two K's in accordance with a general change of German orthography, although in the same paper (with de Lint[28]) the term "Capillar-elektrometrisch" was written with one C and one K. After the construction of the string galvanometer the term electrocardiogram became generally accepted; Einthoven himself then attributed its introduction sometimes to Waller.

---

[a]   In its narrow glass capillary a mercury column borders on a weak solution of sulphuric
      acid: this boundary moves whenever a potential difference between the mercury and the
      acid is applied, changed or removed (fig.3, taken from Einthoven's paper [21]).

Figure 3. *Schematic drawing of the essential part of Lippmann's electrometer.*
A. *Mercury reservoir ending in glass capillary, upper half of which is filled with mercury.* B. *Lower half of capillary and lower reservoir with sulphuric acid. The borderline between mercury and sulphuric acid is not flat but spherical on the side of mercury because of the surface tension which is also responsible for bearing the weight of the mercury column (if not too high; then some mercury spills on the floor)*

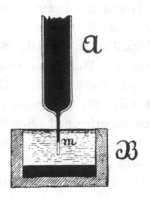

In 1894 the new arrangement was used for the first phonocardiographic tracings in normal persons together with 2 patients suffering from aortic insufficiency[23]. The phonocardiogram was also recorded in rabbits and in a dog with experimental aortic insufficiency. Special attention was paid to the time relations of the electrocardiogram and the phonocardiogram at different sites of the precordium; not to composition or wave frequency of the sound records.

In spite of the marked improvement of the electrocardiographic tracings (fig.4) Einthoven was not satisfied with the shape of them, as they remained disfigured by friction and inertia of the mercury column in the capillary of the Lippmann electrometer (this was also noticed earlier by Waller but apparently accepted as inevitable). Einthoven devised a mathematical correction, which he later found to be similar in effect, although different in method, to the correction earlier proposed by Burch, who worked with Burdon Sanderson at Oxford[24][b].

---

[b] Einthoven referred to Burch in his paper of 1895, but Burdon Sanderson, who probably had not read this paper himself, protested against Einthoven's supposed omission of the work of Burch. This provoked Einthoven to write his first and only public self-defence (Vertheidigung gegen Burdon Sanderson,[26]). Even so, he did not convince Burdon Sanderson; perhaps because both the original article and the defence note were written in German. This annoyed Einthoven very much as appears from his correspondence with Julius. However, after the publication of the string galvanometer Burdon Sanderson was fully interested and Einthoven bore no grudge.

The method of Burch was used for correcting action currents records of skeletal muscle.

To eliminate confusion with the uncorrected tracings and to allow space for possible later additions (such as later actually happened for the U-wave) the letters PQRST from the middle of the alphabet were substituted for ABCD in designing the different peaks in the electrocardiogram (fig.4). With his corrected tracings in hand Einthoven in 1895 began to define the normal electrocardiogram, its variations and subdivisions[24]. For this purpose the phonocardiogram was helpful; for instance, it served well for determining the duration of the systolic period which in the mechanical tracings of the heart beat (cardiogram) was defined very differently by various authors. Einthoven could confirm the earlier finding of Marey that the end of systole coincided with the end of the systolic plateau in the cardiogram.

Standardization of the electrocardiographic method was recognized as a necessity but was carried out gradually in keeping with growing experience and deepening of understanding. In the paper by Einthoven and de Lint (1900)[28] the choice of the standard limb leads was not yet fixed; the division according to Waller in favourable and unfavourable leads (high and low voltage respectively) and the connection with their positioning (across the heart's axis or parallel to it) was confirmed. In the paper of 1900 Einthoven only used a lead from both hands. Some doubt was still present whether the Q wave constituted the end of atrial activity or the beginning of the ventricular complex.

The electrocardiogram at rest and after exertion were compared for the first time, the main purpose being to test the influence of heart rate. Likewise the electrocardiogram was studied in different positions of the body; the exclusive use of lead I allowed conclusions about the change of shape when the ECG was taken in three different horizontal positions: dorsal, right lateral and left lateral respectively. Gauging of voltage had been introduced already in de Vogel's thesis (then expressed in millidaniells, in 1900 in millivolts). The height of individual waves was accurately measured and so was their duration.

Besides the electrocardiogram of normal persons the electrocardiograms were studied from 2 patients with aortic insufficiency, whose phonocardiograms had been published previously. It was found that the T waves were abnormally low in one case, slightly negative in the other.

In the next chapter it will be seen that investigations described in 1900, were later taken up again and extended with the string galvanometer, leading to a fully elaborated system of standardization, complemented with an exploration of abnormal electrocardiograms.

Einthoven's first studies of the electrocardiogram had been possible through technical improvements of the Lippmann electrometer and the circuit in which it had to be incorporated; they were based on physical and mathematical examination of the instrument. Equally important was its protection against mechanical disturbance by the environment (see below). In particular the movement of the mercury column in the capillary demanded more knowledge of mathematics than Einthoven's high school and medical training had provided. He supplemented this mainly through self-study; learning differential and integral calculus from Lorentz' book on the subject in the early 1890's.

30 Years later he presented a copy of this book to Frank Wilson with the words: "May I send you the excellent book of Lorentz' Differential- und Integralrechnung? I have learned my mathematics from it after my nomination as a professor in this University and I hope you will have as much pleasure and profit by it as I have had myself".

In physical matters he was aided by his correspondence and talks with his friend (and later brother-in-law) Julius, who became extra-ordinary professor of physics at Amsterdam and subsequently full professor at Utrecht, where they had studied together.

Figure 4 (opposite page). *Illustration composed from and comparing three subsequent episodes of electrocardiographical development.*

1) Upper part: Waller 1887 [108]. *t=time, h=external pulsation from heartbeat usually called cardiogram (after Marey), e=electrical heart action, showing 2 peaks directed downwards. The cardiac action current is rather inconspicuous and was later often confused with the cardiogram above it.*

2) Einthoven's tracing as published in 1902 [30], *also with Lippmans electrometer. 4 peaks (ABCD) directed upwards because of reversed connection. Timescale in 0,1 sec above tracing.*

Same tracing corrected mathematically. Timescale in 0.1 sec is stretched (S); the 4 peaks in the corrected tracing are now called PQRST.

3) One of the first electrocardiograms with the string galvanometer as published in 1902 [30] *and 1903* [31]. *Timescale with vertical lines at 0.2 sec and dots at 0.04 sec. Like the other electrocardiograms shown above, taken from both hands of Einthoven's chief mechanic van der Woerd.*

1.
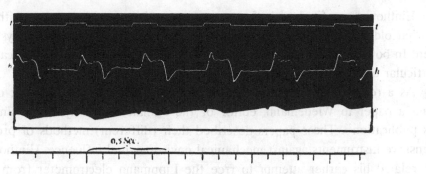

0.5 Sec.

2.
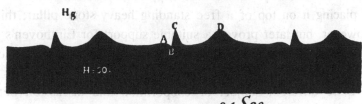

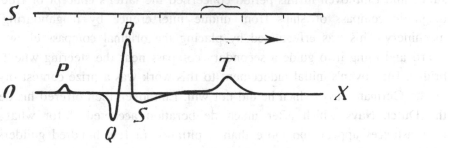

3.
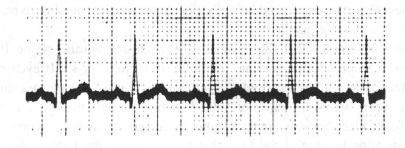

Einthoven profited also from written and personal contact with the somewhat older and already famous Lorentz, professor of theoretical physics at Leiden. In both cases he asked for advice during the preparation of publications, in particular those concerning the Lippmann electrometer.

As a result of the correspondence with Julius, both of them went on by sending a paper to Wiedemann, editor of the Annalen der Physik for simultaneous publication[25]. These papers described their (different) methods of protecting sensitive instruments against mechanical environmental influence. Einthoven's paper related his earlier attempt to free the Lippmann electrometer from such disturbances by placing it on top of a free standing heavy stone pillar; this was not sufficient however, but later proved a suitable support for Einthoven's string galvanometer. In the case of the electrometer it was also necessary to place the instrument on a heavy platform, which floated on mercury.

Another, quite different subject of cooperation and discussion between Julius and Einthoven in this period concerned the latter's concept of freeing the magnetic compass of ships from undue interference by neighbouring heavy machinery. This was effectuated by placing the original compass elsewhere on board and using it to guide a secondary compass near the steering wheel on the bridge. Einthoven's initial inducement to this work was a prize contest organized by the German Navy, which he did not win. Einthoven then offered his design to the Dutch Navy which after much deliberation accepted it for what in the circumstances appears no more than a pittance (a few hundred guilders). The whole series of events, as far as it can be reconstructed from the correspondence, shows Einthoven's perseverance and inventiveness as well as his inability to make financial profit from these qualities.

There is little doubt that Einthoven (fig.5) in the last decade of the 19th century already planned his programme for the next 15 years or so. It even can be shown that Einthoven was aware of the far reaching impact of electrocardiography several years before his paper of 1900.[28] In 1893 he presented to a Dutch medical audience electrocardiography and phonocardiography as new methods of clinical investigation in spite of the fact, that his records of the human electrocardiogram at that moment were far removed from their later state of perfection[21].

His determination is shown in the correspondence with his slightly younger brother Johan who was successfully building a career in the civil service of the Dutch East Indies. This correspondence however, also shows Einthoven's doubt of his own capacities.

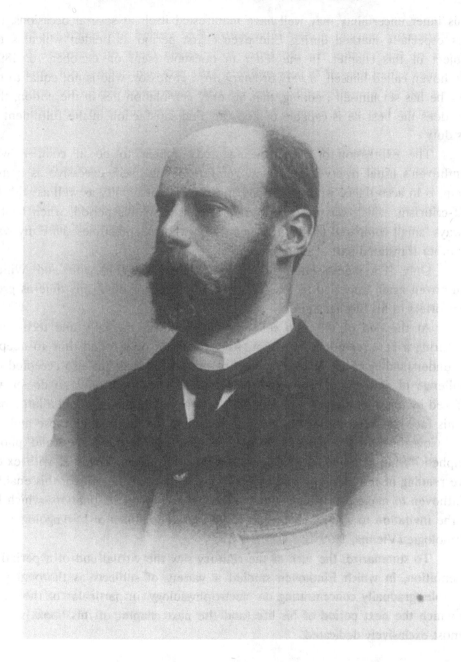

Figure 5.   *Willem Einthoven in his thirties; a period of foresight and determin-ation but also of doubt and uncertainties.*

This inner uncertainty may well have manifested itself at several occasions, but was especially marked during Einthoven's first period at Leiden which is the subject of this chapter. In the letter in question (sent on October 16, 1896) Einthoven called himself "a very ordinary little professor, who is not equal to the task he has set himself"; adding, that his only consolation lies in the notion, that "he does the best he is capable of and can find satisfaction in the fulfilment of his duty".

The expression of these feelings may appear to be in contrast with Einthoven's usual reserved character; yet the feeling itself, excessive as it may seem, is in accordance with his serious and sincere personality as well as with his self-criticism, which was perhaps most pronounced in this period, when he felt always "small compared to the great genii with whom I sometimes share my way" (another translated part of the same letter).

Only five weeks later, his brother Johan lost his wife and Willem Einthoven again appealed to love of work and sense of duty, this time as great comforters in his brother's grief.

At the end of the 19th century, while he was mentally and technically preparing a new recording apparatus, Einthoven not only found time to deepen his understanding of his beloved subject of optical illusions but also accepted the challenge of studying a very different problem. The opportunity to do so was offered by the operation of a patient with orbital carcinoma in whom a large part of his face was removed at the left side including the hard palate, nose and left eye. Consequently the movements of the pharynx could be seen and photographed during acts like speaking, swallowing and suction. Together with extensive reading of the literature and observations on himself in a mirror this enabled Einthoven to make a thorough study of the physiology of the pharynx, which led to the invitation to write a chapter in Heymann's Handbuch of Laryngologie and Rhinologie (Vienna, 1899 [27]).

To summarize: the turn of the century saw the virtual end of a period of orientation, in which Einthoven studied a variety of subjects as thoroughly as possible, gradually concentrating on electrophysiology, in particular of the heart, to which the next period of his life (and the next chapter of this book) will be almost exclusively dedicated.

Chapter three (1901-1915).

The string galvanometer and its applications; development of electrocardiography.

The correction of the Lippmann tracings whereby the true shape of the electrocardiogram was revealed did not constitute an endpoint. The mathematical correction had to be repeated for every tracing and was too cumbersome for widespread clinical use. Einthoven set out to develop an instrument which would be both rapid and sensitive enough to obviate the need of correction. Whereas Lippmann's electrometer was sensitive but too slow, the mirror galvanometer of Deprez-d'Arsonval in which a small moving coil of conducting wire was suspended in a magnetic field was rapid in its recording but not sensitive enough to register the heart's action currents. Starting from the latter type of galvanometer Einthoven calculated the requirements for increasing its sensitivity. He found that reducing the weight of the moving coil and of the number and dimensions of its windings as well as increasing the strength of the magnetic field would be necessary. So he decided to use a single thin and short wire of silver-coated quartz placed in a narrow space between the poles of a strong electro-magnet; each of the poles was perforated by holes through which the string could be illuminated and observed respectively by means of two microscopes; see the schematic illustrations taken from Einthoven's paper:" Le Télécardiogramme" (fig.6a, 6b) and the photographic exterior in fig.7. During the construction of this "string galvanometer" Einthoven became aware of another instrument with a string in a magnetic field, devised by Ader[1] as a receiver of Morse signals transmitted by underseas telegraph cables. It was neither intended nor ever used as a galvanometer, that is for measuring electrical currents. Einthoven duly mentioned its existence in his first publication of the string galvanometer[29]; in the same way he mentioned in a later publication (1909[40]) Ewing's use of an instrument with two strings for measuring magnetic field intensity, prior to Ader[65]. In this paper of 1909 Einthoven also calculated the sensitivity of Ader's radiotelegraphic receiver (if it had been used as a galvanometer) as only 1:100.000 compared to the string galvanometer.

However, Einthoven's mention of Ader's string instrument sometimes led to the impression, that Einthoven's string galvanometer was based on improvement of Ader's "galvanometer" rather than on purposeful research and invention. This will be further discussed in chapter 7 together with the fact that

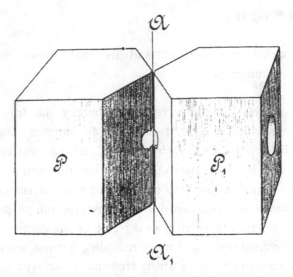

Figure 6a.   *Principle of the string galvanometer as depicted in 2 schematic drawings by Einthoven in "The télécardiogramme" (1906). The poles P and P1 of the electromagnet leave only a narrow space for the string A-A1 to move in and are pierced by holes for the two microscopes (see fig. 6b).*

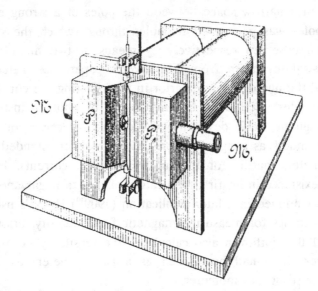

Figure 6b.   *View from above and front. At the right the electromagnet with its poles close to each other and the string in the narrow space in between. Also visible are the two microscopes (resp. for illuminating and observing the string).*

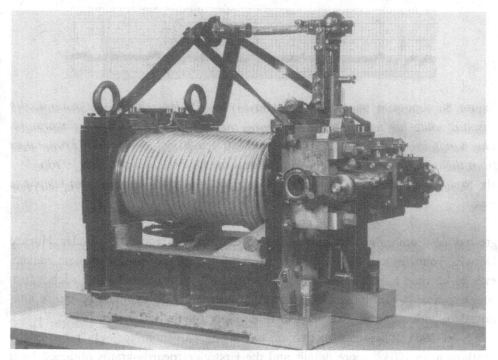

Figure 7   *Finished string galvanometer. The long sides of the magnet are covered together by the windings of the tube for water cooling .*

the manufacturing firm Edelmann used this kind of reasoning as an excuse for suspending a contract (see Barron's booklet[3] and Einthoven's correspondence with father and son Edelmann and their ally Professor Ebert in chapter 7). Privately Einthoven objected a few times gently to colleagues who unintentionally sided with Edelmann in a paper or book by calling Ader's instrument a string galvanometer.

In Med. History[9] Burnett pointed out that Einthoven and subsequently the firms who made commercial types of the string galvanometer used several recently developed materials and methods in order to obtain both high sensitivity and swift response. He also revealed interesting aspects of the scientific back-

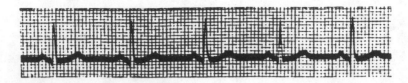

Figure 8a (opposite page) and 8b (above). 8a: *Patient sitting in the university hospital while his telecardiogram is being taken in the physiological laboratory. The hands are immersed in strong salt (NaCl) solution for lead I. (Print taken from the original negative for the illustration in "Le Télécardiogramme" 1906* [33.] 8b: *Result of recording. Note excellent quality of tracing transmitted via telephone wire.*

ground of Cambridge Scientific Instruments, dating from its founder Horace Darwin, youngest son of Charles Darwin and one of the rare instrument makers ever to become a fellow of the Royal Society. It is not surprising that such a firm could understand Einthoven being "more concerned with his integrity and reputation than with money", in contrast to Edelmann (for the latter see chapter 7).

In 1901 [29] the construction of the string galvanometer was reported by Einthoven; in 1903 [31] more details and the first electrocardiograms obtained by it were published. It must have been a great satisfaction to Einthoven, that these tracings equalled the corrected Lippmann tracings, thereby vindicating both his correction method and the string galvanometer. In 1906 the laboratory was connected with the academic hospital - at a distance of a mile - by underground telephone cables intertwined at their free hanging endings. Consequently the first series of "telecardiograms" from patients could be recorded (fig.8a and 8b) and described[33,34] (see chapter 5, section 2 for Bosscha's help and the opportunity, which the simultaneous construction of the Leiden telephone system offered). This was followed in 1908 by a further series of electrocardiographic findings in patients[35]. At this time Einthoven's system of standardization was completed, which was soon adopted almost universally (with the exception of Waller and Nicolai who defended their own systems of leads respectively denomination, see chapters 6 and 7).

Most abnormal findings concerned rhythm disturbances: various grades of heart block (also studied experimentally by vagal stimulation), ventricular extrasystoles, atrial flutter and fibrillation; the latter two were not yet understood

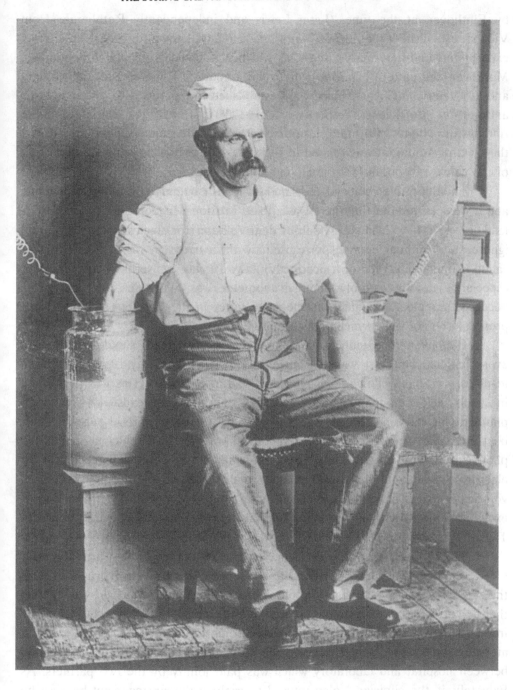

by Einthoven at the time. (Later Lewis and independently Rothberger from Vienna established the identity with the already known disorders in animal experiments and veterinary disease, as will be discussed in chapter 6, section 3). Moreover, the pattern of atrial hypertrophy (enlarged P wave) and that of right and left ventricular hypertrophy, were established in patients with mitral stenosis and aortic insufficiency respectively. In 1908 [35] Einthoven confirmed these findings in patients with mitral insufficiency and aortic stenosis, pointing out that the electrocardiogram was related to the state of the cardiac muscle, not to that of the valves responsible for the altered hemodynamics.

The definitive choice of the standard leads currently still in use, was made and it was pointed out that there was a fixed relation between them, expressed as lead II - lead I = lead III. A self-evident relation for a closed circuit, if one ignores the minimal energy loss caused by the current in the string. This was called Einthoven's rule or (incorrectly) law. It was a useful check however, especially as long as only one galvanometer was available for registration, because the peaks designated by the same letter in the different standard leads proved to be not quite synchronous.

Einthoven repeatedly stressed, that at least two leads should be taken in every patient. The best way of course was to simultaneously register all three leads (or two pairs of two leads with one lead in common). This was performed in a later stage (see pp. 99 and 117 and fig.22) but different leads with a common photographic reference tracing like a mechanical record of carotid pulse or heart beat etc. were often used before that time. However, in Einthoven's hands the phonocardiogram provided the best information in relating mechanical to electrical myocardial activity. The abnormal shape of the QRS complex in ventricular extrasystoles was explained by an abnormal pathway of the spread of excitation, while the concept of the normal pathway was brought into line with Tawara's description of the conducting system published in 1906.[106]

The cooperation of the clinician Nolen at Leiden was luke-warm and after a few years came to an end, when the connection was broken. It was said later that the clinician resented that the physiologist sometimes reported by telephone that he could see an extrasystole before the clinician could feel the corresponding intermission of the pulse (de Waart[108]). According to Fahr[67] however the immediate cause of disagreement concerned the cost of maintenance of the connection between hospital and laboratory which was paid jointly by the two partners. As Fahr tells it, the clinician Nolen refused to prolong this arrangement because he felt that all the credit was going to Einthoven and that he was not even getting honourable mention. Einthoven on the other hand, Fahr said, was not prepared to pay Nolen's half because he felt sure, that "Nolen will ultimately make money out of it, people demand an electrocardiogram". [a]

It is also clear from Fahr's account that he would have loved to start a clinical unit in the hospital in collaboration with Einthoven's laboratory and his galvanometer, but this opportunity never materialized. This matter will be discussed again in chapter 6 (section 1 about Fahr). It is certain that the lack of a cooperating clinician must have been a handicap and sometimes perhaps a painful experience, but there is no record that Einthoven ever showed such feelings either publicly or privately. Even though university and faculty matters often occasioned contact between Einthoven and Nolen, who was the former's successor as rector of the university and as dean of the medical faculty (both times after having been secretary under Einthoven's presidency). Addresses directed by Einthoven to Nolen at formal meetings and celebrations are on record in abstract; they never refer to electrocardiography but occasionally to Nolen's knowledge and love of Greek.

In 1908 however Thomas Lewis, a young clinician at University College of London, having studied arrhythmias by Mackenzie's method of venous and arterial pulse records, sent a letter asking for a reprint of "Le Télécardiogramme" (Einthoven's paper on the electrocardiogram of patients mentioned above[33]). From then on a long lasting correspondence (fully published in 1983)[102] and a growing contact between Lewis and Einthoven with several mutual visits followed, which proved of great value both to the correspondents and to electrocardiography. The two men soon learned to respect and appreciate each other; they displayed similar qualities of persevering search for the solution of problems and at the same time a divergence of interests and abilities which were more or less complementary. Einthoven the physiologist with a marked general concern about patients and general medicine was at heart a physicist though not by training and office, as A.V. Hill later (1927[70]) pointed out and Lewis was a clinician also trained as a physiologist, who was very effective in devising appropriate experi-

---

[a] Einthoven's prophecy (as quoted by Fahr) did not come true, if one may judge from Nolen's valedictory address in 1924. [94] There it becomes clear, that for Nolen the inventions of Röntgen and Einthoven deserved admiration but only occasionally a clinical application (quoting Mackenzie and contending that too many new methods were being introduced).In contrast, Nolen emphasized the importance of a broad classical education (including Latin and Greek) of every physician in order to improve his understanding of the patient's needs.

ments for the solution of clinical problems. There was a tacit understanding on the delineation and independence of their respective fields and on the other hand a mutual interest in the other's work and readiness to give information. This was especially noticeable when Lewis, whose knowledge of physics and mathematics was rather limited as he himself realised, approached Einthoven with questions on physical aspects. On the other hand Einthoven did not pursue any investigation which Lewis had already tackled or which required clinical experience. Moreover Einthoven was fairly often confronted with other problems, which were not or only indirectly related to electrocardiography but evoked his interest enough to justify further study. In part these problems were purely physical or technical, but relevant to electro-physiological research.

In other, less frequent, instances Einthoven's attention was drawn to problems of a different nature, such as for instance the psycho-galvanic reflex, which in turn led to a study of skin resistance and polarization as well as further research on electrical conduction in the body (see chapter 4, page 47). When at another occasion Einthoven was asked by a court of justice to give evidence about the amount of dexterity involved in a particular game which might be interpreted as an unlawful game of hazard, this led to a study (and a paper) on the precision of movements of the hand. Such subjects were not mentioned to Lewis, although most reprints were sent to him.

As a rule this arrangement worked well. The instances in which it did not forestall misunderstandings or where another course could have yielded better results, were rare; one of these will be discussed in chapter 6, section 3. The influence of Einthoven on Lewis was recognized by the latter on several occasions, most clearly perhaps in 1911 by the dedication of his book "The mechanism of the heart beat"[87] to both Mackenzie and Einthoven, the two men who guided Lewis' career to a certain extent in successive phases of his life. Mackenzie particularly in the beginning, but again later, when Lewis terminated his work on electrocardiography and certainly also during World War I when Lewis was assigned to study the "soldier's heart syndrome" under Mackenzie's (also Osler's and Clifford Albutt's) supervision. In between, it was often Einthoven to whom Lewis turned for information and guidance when he felt the need of it.

In 1912 Einthoven was invited by the Chelsea Clinical Society, a local association of practitioners at London, to give a lecture. Through Lewis' efforts and his appeal to Mackenzie and Osler (particularly the latter had means and influence) the occasion acquired a much greater importance. It was completed by a meeting of the Royal Society of Medicine on the clinical use of the electrocardiogram, where Einthoven gave a short introductory address published in the proceedings of this meeting. His Chelsea lecture anticipated his paper on the equilateral triangle, which will be discussed below. Einthoven's Chelsea lecture itself was very soon published in the Lancet[43] (but not quite to his satisfaction, as he wrote to Lewis).

Einthoven kept some notes of this trip to London, which were found in a book of his library. They were kindly shown to me by the Leiden physiologist Professor Tammeling and constitute a very detailed account of Einthoven's modest expenses together with a dry, matter-of-fact report on little events. No doubt he will have used them for humorous tales at home: a president who had forgotten Einthoven's name, an important guest who slept during Einthoven's speech and another who commented on Einthoven's lecture by saying that the dinner afterwards was much easier to digest.

The last remark deserved more praise for candour than for politeness; however, on reading the paper in the Lancet again, it must be admitted that Einthoven in his Chelsea lecture probably overestimated the understanding of a great part of his audience. The following year he elaborated and rewrote the paper mentioning cooperation of Fahr and de Waart[46]. This time many illustrations and especially the appendix clarify the rather complicated web of theoretical considerations and their practical application. This dualism led to a lengthy title [b] and the introduction therein of a new term, the "manifest potential". This term is defined in the text in a purely mathematical fashion; in the appendix its etymological explanation becomes clarified: i.e. that part of the cardiac potential which you can lay your hands on (Einthoven did not use this unscientific expression, but probably he meant just that). In this particular context the term can be specified as: that part of the cardiac vector, which can be measured (or rather constructed) from the standard leads (see below).

To give a brief summary of Einthoven's simplifying scheme: the heart is represented as the centre of an equilateral triangle (the "body", in fact an electrically homogeneous sheet in its frontal plane) with the standard leads on its sides. The heart's electric force arises through summation of all the potential differences of the active parts of the heart muscle. The size and direction of the resulting potential difference can be represented by a vector originating in the

---

[b] In its English translation (Hoff and Sekelj, 1950 [47]) the title reads: " On the direction and manifest size of the variation of potential in the human heart and on the influence of the position of the heart on the form of the electrocardiogram".

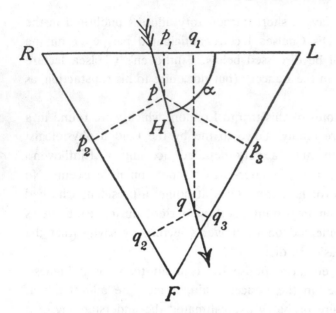

Figure 9. *Scheme of equi-lateral triangle. The summated potential differ-ence is the distance p - q on the heart vector H at a given instant with its direc-tion (angle α).*
The deflections in the three standard leads (Lead I = R - L arm, Lead II = R arm - foot, Lead III = foot - L arm) are the pro-jections of p - q on the three sides of the triangle.

centre of the triangle; it can be constructed from its projections on the sides of the triangle which equal the simultaneous deflections in the respective leads (fig.9). This heart vector (or electrical axis) changes at every instance in size and direction due to a) the progression of the cardiac activation and b) the influence of the heart's position which varies with the position of the body [c] and also with (deep) respiration. In passing Einthoven remarks also that the vector which represents a potential difference, must originate in two points lying close to each other (i.e. a bipole or dipole, but Einthoven does not use that term here). The choice of the equilateral triangle for this scheme was explained by Einthoven to Lewis in a letter (see below and chapter 6 section 3).

This paper of 1913 [46,47] has always been one of Einthoven's best known and most influential papers; vectorcardiography derives from it. Nevertheless it has often been misunderstood, particularly by those who mistook the simplified scheme for reality or who thought that Einthoven himself confused the two. Careful reading of the paper would have shown that this interpretation is wrong.

---

[c]   The infrequent but instructive situation of situs cordis inversus causing an upside down image of the electrocardiogram in lead I and exchange of the usual leads II and III was already reported by Waller in 1889 [110]. It was also described by Einthoven in the paper discussed here [46] and reiterated in an addendum to a paper by Gorter in Acta Paediatriaca (1925 [58])

A study comparing the electrical axis and the anatomical axis as determined by fluoroscopy, later showed that they are not identical (as Waller assumed in 1889 [111]) but that changes in direction are practically the same in both cases. Flohil's thesis[68] about these findings was only published after Einthoven's death.

Vectorcardiography on the other hand started already during Einthoven's lifetime with Mann's method of "monocardiography" of 1920 [92], in which the successive endpoints of Einthoven's electrical vector are joined to a curve. In the same year Fahr[66] used the direction of successive electrical vectors to challenge Lewis' terminology of bundlebranch block. Lewis dismissed Fahr's objections and Einthoven perhaps had Fahr in mind, when he spoke of theoretical objections made against Lewis' theory; at any rate, he did not support Fahr (see also chapter 6, section 1). Neither did Einthoven (or Flohil for that matter), discuss Mann's paper on the monocardiogram[92].

In 1912 Einthoven wrote his first review of electro-cardiography called: "Über die Deutung des Electrokardiogramms" (on the explanation of the electrocardiogram[42]). Two major aspects stand out:

1) In discussing the opinion of other authors Einthoven consistently opposes the view that the deflections of the ventricular complex indicate the (changing) direction of the excitatory wave. This stand he maintained throughout his life, although he later made a partial exception for Lewis' theory of the biventricular origin of the QRS complex (which seemed to be based on irrefutable anatomical, experimental and pathological evidence, but led to an erroneous nomenclature of bundlebranch block pattern, see discussion in chapter 6 section 3).

2) At the end of his paper Einthoven warns against impatience because of the still unknown basic origin and significance of the electrocardiographic deflections. He contends that the importance of a full explanation should not be overestimated and points out which findings had already come to light so far (atrial and ventricular part of the electrocardiogram, atrioventricular block, unilateral hypertrophy particularly of the ventricles etc.). More insight into Einthoven's view on electrocardiography had already been revealed in an address to his university of Leiden (see end of this chapter).

A topic in the field of circulatory dynamics was examined with Korteweg in 1915 [48]: the variability of the pulse in auricular fibrillation. In this paper the influence of the variations in aortic pressure causing changes in resistance to ventricular ejection, was pointed out in addition to the effect of varying cardiac filling and corresponding output which had already been noted in the literature.

Closer to electrocardiography, the study of heart sounds was taken up again and extended this time using the string galvanometer, as published by Battaerd in Heart[4]. A third sound, already heard by Gibson on auscultation, was recorded and described by Einthoven with Wieringa and Snijders[36].

A different subject altogether was the electrical reaction of the eye's retina to light, as a rule examined in isolated frog's eyes. The first measurements of this kind in Einthoven's laboratory were carried out by de Haas (with the rather insensitive Deprez-d'Arsonval galvanometer) and described in his thesis of 1903[69]. The main conclusion of de Haas was that Fechner's law (arithmetical increase of stimulus strength causes geometrical progression of effect) could be confirmed for stimuli of medium strength in the excised frog's eye, i.e. without interference of the brain.

In 1908 new research on this topic was carried out by Einthoven and Jolly with the string galvanometer[37]; it showed a composite action curve, which on analysis seemed to be due to three separate functions (or substances). It took several decades more before the electroretinogram was applied in the clinic; altogether 100 years or so after the eye's electrical reaction was first reported by Holmgren in 1865.

Einthoven and Jolly's work however served as a starting point for further research in the 1920's (Adrian and Matthews) and 1930's (Granit). A.D. Waller came to Leiden in 1909 to study again the effect of slight massage of the eyeball which he had previously described. Westerlund from Sweden, who without success had tried to register retinal currents also came to profit from the string galvanometer at Leiden, which for several decades was the best and for some years even the only reliable instrument available for studying weak electrical action currents. They were among the first visitors who were allowed to work with the string galvanometer.

Furthermore, it should be mentioned that in this extraordinary fertile period of research Einthoven also studied the relationship of vagal nerve and heart. In 1908[38,39] he published with Flohil and Battaerd records of the centripetal vagal action currents after cutting the nerve in the neck and compensating for the demarcation current. The vagal action currents in the dog proved to consist of a superposition of a continuous series of frequent and small waves upon a similar series of slower and larger waves. Earlier Lewandowsky used already a Deprez-d'Arsonval galvanometer in 1898 and Alcode and Sperman in 1905 a Lippmann capillary electrometer to register vagal action currents. They found waves that proved to be related to change of lung volume. Einthoven confirmed this for the large waves he had found and moreover showed that on inflating the lungs and sucking them out, the effects of inflation are more easily exhausted by fatigue and injury than those of evacuation. He supposed this difference to be due to the existence of two different sets of fibres. The rapid and small waves in the vagogram proved to be due to the stimulation of the depressor nerve, which in the dog (and also in man) is incorporated into the vagus nerve, but remains independent in the rabbit, causing the two sets of waves to appear separately in the latter animal (in the vagus and the depressor nerve respectively). With respect to man Einthoven pointed out two possible implications of the proximity between these two nerves: 1) the virtually fixed relation between heart rate and respiratory frequency which had been known already for a long time; 2) that vagal tone is probably maintained by the action of the heart.

As a counterpart to this research Einthoven (with Wieringa) had published in 1911[44,45] various centrifugal vagal effects on the heart as shown by the electrocardiogram, some of which (e.g. A.V.block) he had already published. The variable effect of vagal stimulation (electrically of the nerve itself or by intravenous injection of morphine which excites the vagal centre in the medulla oblongata) proved to differ in various parts of the heart and also to depend on the strength of the electrical stimulus respectively dosage of morphine. Experimentally the latter had an inverse effect in very high doses by increasing heart rate instead of slowing it.

Einthoven's activities outside his laboratory and his home, where he also spent much time on planning his work and writing it up, were very limited as far as leisure is concerned (this included his formerly favourite sport except for hours of skating in the winter (Fahr), when the ice was sufficiently strong). Every year during three weeks in July the laboratory was closed however and Einthoven then had to postpone work and the reception of visitors. During these periods as transpires from the correspondence, Einthoven and his family often went to live at the Dutch seaside in the neighbourhood of Leiden, or in the woods further east; at least as long as the children were young.

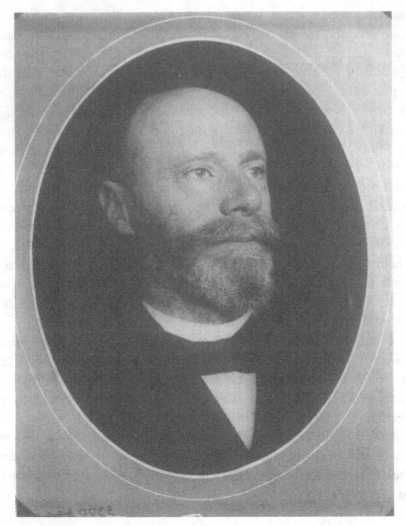

Figure 10.   *Willem Einthoven when rector of the senate in 1906 (in his most fruitful period and more sure of himself than a decade ago).*

Trips abroad were virtually confined to attendance of international congresses and occasionally invited lectures; Einthoven's American lecturing tour will be discussed in chapter 4.

Many interested scientists from abroad wanted to see the string galvanometer or asked permission for themselves or for their collaborators to work with it. From the correspondence it is clear that another, larger group only asked for information, photographs of records, reprints, etc. All were courteously answered, while only in a few cases these contacts were of advantage to Einthoven himself; Lewis was a fortunate exception. After Einthoven's death it was mentioned in several obituaries, that while receiving visitors or meeting other scientists at congresses, Einthoven's attitude was always friendly and obliging, irrespective of the age and position of his interlocutor.

It is characteristic for Einthoven's sense of duty (and perhaps also his desire of a broad point of view) that he almost never failed to appear at the regular meetings of the university, medical faculty or Royal Academy of Sciences (of which he was a member since 1902 and where his participation in the discussion on widely diverging subjects was highly appreciated). This habit was maintained until his final illness and was praised by the medical faculty's dean, who upheld Einthoven, then the oldest member of the faculty, as an example to his younger colleagues because he was the only one who had never been absent from faculty meetings during the current term. As mentioned earlier in this chapter Einthoven became in due course rector of the university (and 2 years before that dean of the faculty) for a year, according to custom.

As rector (fig.10), Einthoven delivered a speech in 1906 reviewing the development and significance of electrophysiology, in particular electrocardiography, without mentioning that most of the work had been carried out in his own laboratory. Einthoven made it clear that the chemical changes, from which the action currents must be supposed to originate, were unknown so far but that registration of the electric activity of organs is of fundamental importance as an objective and measurable evidence of the function of these organs. As a matter of fact, this was an elaboration of an earlier statement made in his inaugural address of 1886, i.e. that the action current is a "symbol of activity". De Waart[108] also recalls this initial notion but relates it to the question of the synchronism of mechanical and electrical activity of the myocardium, repeatedly studied by Einthoven and co-workers in the period of 1916 through 1924 and discussed in chapter 4. Both historical associations lead to the same conclusion, i.e that Einthoven's mind often harboured ideas for many years before he presented them in a final form or published the pertinent investigations. This conclusion was also drawn by de Waart (l.c.) who cited other instances of this practice.

Chapter four (1916-1927).

Ultimate improvement of the string galvanometer; its achievements and limitations. Einthoven's American lecture tour and Nobel Prize. Survey of electrocardiography completed during final illness.

In his last period Einthoven was able to perfect his string galvanometer and to increase its sensitiveness to the utmost, while further exploring its usefulness in various directions; some of them new, others dating from earlier phases of his career.

Little of this last period in Einthoven's research was directly related to electrocardiography. Three possible reasons for this may be considered:

1) Einthoven had no connection with patients in the hospital any more, although it is true that fairly regularly he made electrocardiograms of patients sent to him by their physicians (in 1932 I saw some of these records and notes in the physiological laboratory, but they have disappeared except one: number 632 of Feb 22nd, 1922). Einthoven also made a chest X-ray of every patient and listened to the heart sounds. He received information about the patient and pointed out what required clinical attention. On March 2, 1919 however he mentioned in a letter to his son, that he went to see a young patient with serious heart disease after urgent request of the father. Obviously this was an exceptional event.

2) In 1925 or thereabouts Lewis terminated his research in electrocardiography. The reason for Lewis' decision is not clear; some possibilities will be dealt with in chapter 6. At any rate, there are indications in Lewis' correspondence with Einthoven, that the former's change of research had not been planned long beforehand. After his own visit to Leiden in April 1921 (his last as it turned out (fig.11) Lewis sent his assistant Drury to Leiden in the fall of 1921 because Lewis wanted him "to become more expert on the electrical and physical side than I have been able to become". Thereafter Lewis wrote on Jan. 5, 1922 to Einthoven: ---"I am extremely grateful for what you have done for him, as I am sure it will not only stand Drury in good stead, but that it will much facilitate the future work in this laboratory". Yet on May 1st. 1926 Lewis wrote:" It is some time now that I have touched the galvanometer, as I have been working at skin circulation that has long interested me".

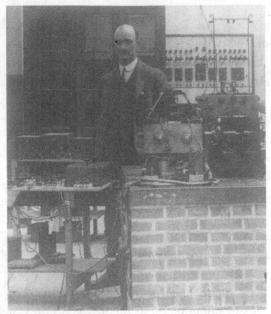

To Mrs. Lewis with kindest
regards from the Leyden friends
of Prof Thomas Lewis
April 1921

Figure 11. *Thomas Lewis' last visit to Leiden; he is seen standing behind a pillar with (presumably) the latest type of string galvanometer on it. The dedication to Mrs Lewis was written by Einthoven.*

Lewis then goes on with questions about the electrical resistance of the skin; in his answer Einthoven offers to send reprints, but it appears that Lewis had received them already: Einthoven's paper with Bijtel on conduction of electrical currents in the human body, (1923 [53]) and that with Roos on skin resistance and potential difference during the psycho-galvanic reflex (1921[51]) Apparently Lewis had not paid attention to them. Einthoven did not complain about Lewis' defection from electrocardiography; he wrote how good it was to have had "the opportunity to say in my Stockholm lecture what I think of your work. I hope you will have the same success with the skin". What Einthoven had said about Lewis at Stockholm was: "It is my conviction that the general interest in electrocardiography would not have risen so high, nowadays, if we had to do without his work and I doubt whether without his valuable contribution I would have the privilege of standing before you today".

3) Perhaps the most important reason for Einthoven to refrain from personal research in clinical electrocardiography after having demonstrated its promising features, may have been his tacit but firm and often apparent guideline not to enter into any research, where he could not - for lack of time, experience or suitable methods - go to the bottom of the problem quantitatively as far as

possible. As long as Lewis was engaged in research on electrocardiography this also included an equally tacit but clear understanding that Einthoven would not take up projects, which were part of Lewis' programme. In the period 1916-1927 discussed here this became noticeable in the matter of bundlebranch block terminology which will be discussed later (chapter 6, section 3).

During World War I and its aftermath, Einthoven's attention was mainly focused on finding new applications for his galvanometer and improving its sensitivity. The most urgent problem at that moment seemed to be the use of the string galvanometer as a receiver of radiotelegrams. His son who studied electrical engineering at Delft, there met director de Groot of the radiotelegraphic laboratory of the Dutch East Indies and discussed with him the idea of using the string galvanometer as a receiver of radiotelegrams. Einthoven Jr proposed to increase the galvanometer's sensitivity not only by further reduction of length and diameter of the string but also by placing it in a vacuum. In fact the concept of a vacuum had been proposed to Willem Einthoven already in the first years of his work with the string galvanometer (by Bosscha, see chapter 5, section 2); furthermore the use of the string galvanometer as a receiver of telegrams (then sent by cable from distant places e.g. across the Atlantic Ocean) also had been suggested by Bosscha when he told Einthoven about a possibility of obtaining a grant for the development of the latter's new instrument. At that time Einthoven himself preferred his project for connecting his laboratory to the academic hospital.

But the present situation was different: radiotelegraphy was available since the beginning of the 20th century but on its long way from the tropics (some 12.000 KM) the signal had to be reinforced a few times at ground stations which were situated on foreign soil, dominated by Great Britain. The latter country was involved in World War I, while Holland remained neutral. Therefore a direct reception in Holland of radiotelegraphic messages from the station on Java was both politically highly desirable and technically a tempting challenge. There may have been hope of a financial reward - from a letter of Willem Einthoven to his son it is clear that they had agreed to share possible profits - but this was surely a secondary consideration.

Einthoven was not a person who could find his way to financial gain from inventions as had become clear at earlier occasions (cf. his invention of a secondary ship's compass and his failed arrangement with Edelmann, mentioned in chapters 2 and 7 respectively). When Drury, assistant to Lewis, came to work with Einthoven and found the laboratory doors closed to him on Fridays, he suspected commercial secrets, according to Kekwick[78] in his obituary of (then) Sir Alan Drury for the Royal Society, but in all probability there was political secrecy involved because of the war situation mentioned above. This was confirmed in a letter from Einthoven to his son then working on Java, in which he deplored the fact that his brother Emile, civil servant in the Dutch East Indies, had received a telegram from Einthoven Sr to Einthoven Jr and reported its arrival with its contents to the family in Holland. Although these contents were innocent enough, they related to the secret development of radiotelegraphic reception arranged with the Dutch government and henceforth everything connected with it had to be kept away from Emile.

In any case, the vacuum string galvanometer was constructed at Leiden and functioned well, except that full use of its increased sensitivity in a virtually complete vacuum was prevented by the occurrence of unrest of the string due to Brownian movements of remaining molecules from the residual air. The latter made the string oscillate in its own frequency if the circuit was open but irregularly if the vacuum was slightly diminished or the circuit was closed and the magnetic field activated[63]. In 1917 Einthoven's son deferred the end of his studies for a year or two and went to work in Java's radiotelegraphic laboratory, taking the new galvanometer with him on board of a Dutch ship, which arrived safely.

The letters of father Einthoven often with additions by mother Einthoven, to their son were preserved in part by the widow of Einthoven Jr and are now kept in the Einthoven archive of the Museum Boerhaave. They show parental solicitude but also scientific and technical worries (see chapter 5, section 7). After a few years of hard work the emission of radiotelegrams could be received by the string galvanometer in the vicinity of the station on Java, but not in Holland. Einthoven Jr came back to Holland to finish his studies. His father did not give up however and was freed from his duties for some months in order to study the problems of radiotransmission. In the meantime Marconi himself and others had already tried without success to use the string galvanometer (an earlier type of course) as a receiver for transatlantic radiotelegraphy. The principal result of Einthoven's studies was his finding that the frequency of the emitted waves should constantly be in strict consonance with the string's own frequency in order to ensure a good reception. This was accomplished and proved successful. A report on this work was written by Einthoven Jr and presented by Einthoven Sr to the Royal Dutch Academy of Sciences in 1923 [62].

A remarkable achievement, but in fact rather belated for two reasons:

1) the war was over and so was the urgent need for independent reception and 2) still more important, the progress of radioemission with high frequencies and its reception could solve the technical problems much sooner than anticipated by Einthoven and many others. As a matter of fact, the report of the Dutch laboratory of radiotelegraphy in 1929 (two years after Einthoven's death) makes it clear that the work with the string galvanometer had been a short-lived episode, although according to de Waart there still was at that time a string galvanometer stationed in the radiotelegraphic laboratory.

In several instances of fundamental research on myocardial function and electrophysiology Einthoven studied the relation of action current and muscular contraction. This started in 1916 [49] with Einthoven's repetition and critical examination of an experiment by Gaskell, who had claimed that in the tortoise heart after elimination of sinus rhythm and lesion of the ventricular apex, vagal stimulation evokes a decrease of the demarcation current, signifying an opposite electrical activity to that which muscular activity would have caused. Moreover, apart from the direction of the current, no electrical activity at all was expected in the first place, because the heart stood still for some time after the sinus rhythm had stopped. Some physiologists suspected an anabolic effect of vagal stimulation to explain these findings. Now the anabolic or in general, the metabolic effect of nerve action on organs was one of the topics which in the course of the 19th century were disputed repeatedly; for example, the direct action of the nerves on heat production was refuted by Claude Bernard and replaced by the notion of indirect action via regulation of local blood supply through vasomotor influence.

To Einthoven however, the unbreakable connection of electrical with mechanical activity of the myocardium was essential because this concerned the clinical relevance of the electrocardiogram, see also section 5 of chapter 6. With his usual accuracy he set out to follow every step in Gaskell's technique, trying to find an explanation for the unexpected and to Einthoven implausible, result. It became clear that during vagal stimulation a contraction of the lungs occurred, whereby the atrium was stretched because it was fixed by a thread to a pole while it rested on top of the pericardium. The latter moved with every change of lung volume, which could easily be proven by inflating and deflating the lungs. It was this stretching of the auricle in Gaskell's experiment which caused a change of potential and of demarcation current.

During the following years Einthoven disproved many other apparent signs of dissociation between electrical and mechanical activity of the myocardium (which used to be explained by a supposed linkage of electrical activity to stimulation rather than to contraction of the myocardium). Einthoven pointed out the great difference in sensitivity between the methods used for recording the electrical and the mechanical effects respectively. Together with his staff (fig.12) he showed repeatedly the virtually complete synchronism of mechanical and electrical myocardial activity by a more sensitive method to register the former, that is, by using a quartz string as mechanical transmitter of movements. The clearest and most convincing account of this problem was given by Einthoven in his 1924 Harvey Lecture at New York [57].

This Harvey lecture formed part of Einthoven's lecture tour in the United States, which he made in the fall of 1924 (fig.13). The tour was organized by H.B. Williams from New York and Einthoven's former assistant George Fahr from Minneapolis as a sequel to the (first) Dunham Lectures which Einthoven delivered at Boston. Between the beginning at Boston and the end at New York Einthoven's tour included Minneapolis and Ann Arbor as well as Cleveland; his audiences consisted usually of hospital staff and other interested doctors, but occasionally only of students and once (at Minneapolis) of physicists and engineers. The tour was an impressive manifestation of international respect for Einthoven, the more so as the announcement of his Nobel Prize appeared in the American press while Einthoven was in the U.S.A. At first he did not accept any congratulations, because he did not believe the news until he obtained confirmation.

The American tour was gratifying moreover in showing to Einthoven the daily and virtually ubiquitous use of the string galvanometer in hospitals and its growing diagnostic value, e.g. in the recognition of coronary thrombosis (myocardial infarct). The latter could be diagnosed from the E.C.G. even by laboratory technicians, as Einthoven saw to his surprise in Sam Levine's department in Boston. Einthoven's astonishment must have been due as Levine supposed [84], to the fact that he was unaware, together with many others in Europe, of the recent developments in America concerning the clinical diagnosis of coronary thrombosis. The latter was shown for instance by the following: when writing about Einthoven's Nobel Prize, Schott stated in the Münchener Med. Wochenschrift of 1925 [99], that with respect to clinical problems a stagnation ("ein gewisser Stillstand") of electrocardiography had taken place in the last few years.

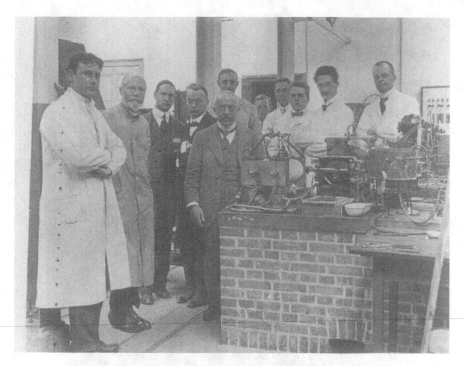

Figure 12.   *Einthoven's co-workers and guests from abroad in the early 1920's. From L. to R.: Bijtel, Einthoven, Verzar(?) (Hungary), Lilienstrand (Stockholm), Bergansius, unknown person at the back, Hoogerwerf, van Lawick van Pabst, van der Bijl, Hugenholtz, de Jongh. The latter had been assistant shortly after 1900 but now had returned in order to prepare his thesis on the time relations of electro- and mechanocardiogram (presented in 1923, when de Jongh was chief of the municipal internal department at the Hague and also personal physician to Queen Wilhelmina). String galvanometer stands on brick pillar; tubing for watercooling and microscope with photographic equipment are visible on the left part of the pillar.*

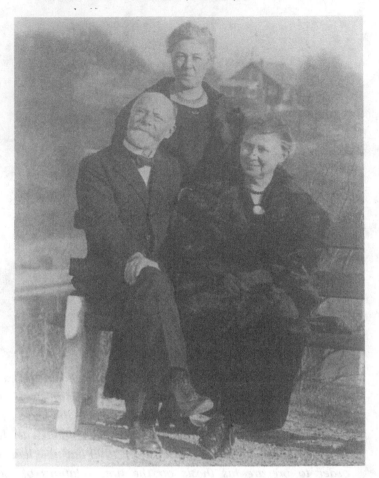

Figure 13.   *The Einthoven's in 1924. Standing behind them Mrs Einthoven's sister, Mrs de Voogd, who joined them on their journey to America. For the two ladies this was chiefly an independent trip. Einthoven in his happy old age.*

Many other honours came to him in this last period such as the foreign membership of the Royal Society and a doctorate honoris causa of Edinburgh as a special feature of the international congress of physiology there in 1923.

However, one of the very first distinctions (in 1913) may have pleased him most, although he hardly wrote or talked about it. This was an honorary degree in physics from his old university of Utrecht where he already had earned his doctor's degree in medicine. It was conferred on him by his brother-in-law, old comrade and friend Julius, now professor of physics at Utrecht.

A phenomenon for which the string galvanometer for a while provided the only possible way of recording, was that of the action currents of the sympathetic nerve. As in Einthoven's previous work on the centripetal impulses of the vagal nerve, time relations were studied in particular. Einthoven's research started after two urgent requests of neurophysiologists, i.e. Byrne from New York and Karplus with Kreidl from Vienna respectively. The first investigation, for which Byrne had brought an operated cat in a basket, was carried out before the construction of the vacuum string galvanometer was completed. When the experiments were published in 1923 [54], it was mentioned that the string had been loosened in order to increase its sensitivity; as a result the accuracy of its tracings had suffered. It could clearly be shown however that irritation by sound or heat as well as electrical stimulation of the ischiadic nerve provoked an action current in the main sympathetic nerve of the cat's neck, which is embedded in a common trunk with the vagus and the depressor nerve. (The latter two show the waves discussed in chapter 3, which are synchronous with respiration and heart beat respectively). The sympathetic action currents leading to different organs (e.g. salivary glands, pupils, etc.) proved to vary in latent period and sometimes in shape.

Karplus and Kreidl wanted to study the effect of hypothalamic stimulation on the sympathetic nerve. In fact a distinct action current in the latter could be demonstrated with the vacuumtype of string galvanometer [60]. However, finer details in the pattern of the nervous impulses did not come to light; here again technical advances (electronic amplification) later provided a better and simpler solution. As mentioned before, Einthoven had already become aware of this possibility around 1920 and had tried with the help of his son to increase the string galvanometer's sensitivity by subsequent electronic amplification. At that time he found the technique unreliable and insufficient. Therefore he became sceptical about later trials (de Waart 1957 [108]) and hoped that improving the string galvanometer itself would sufficiently enhance its sensitivity. A few years

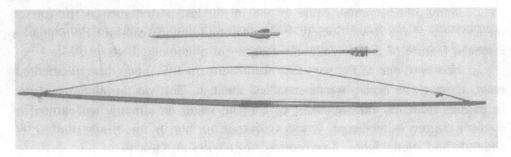

Figure 14. *The bow and arrows which were used to shoot away thin threads of quartz.*

after Einthoven's death, in the 1930's, the work of Adrian and others showed that electronic technique opened the way to great scientific advances in nerve electrophysiology.

A very different use of an extremely thin and short string was that as a mechanical receptor of air vibrations due to the sound of tuning forks or the human voice. It turned out that very high frequencies could be registered: above 15.000 p. sec, nearly the double of the highest limit formerly attained by the combination of microphone and string galvanometer [55,56]. Records of singing showed many harmonics. Interestingly enough, singers often thought to sing at the octave (i.e. the double frequency) of the basic pitch they produced in reality; no doubt due to the greater sensitivity of the human ear for higher overtones, as Einthoven pointed out.

It is evident, that the technical difficulties of manufacturing the strings increased with diminishing dimensions. The strings were still quartz filaments, made as in the beginning by melting pieces of quartz which were shot away; for a long time this was performed with arrow and bow (fig.14). Subsequently the quartz filaments were made conductive by coating them with silver (or gold, which is a better conductor). The final solution for this procedure was to spray the quartz threads in a vacuum, while they were revolved vertically to avoid inequalities.

Figure 15. *One of the last pictures of Einthoven. His signature can be seen with difficulty against the background of the dark chair.*

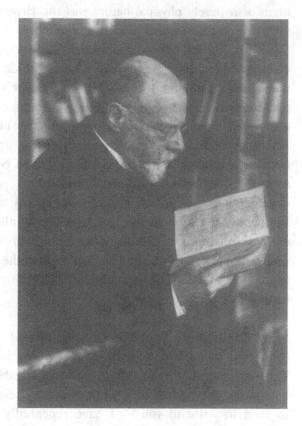

All this took place in a "dust free" room where usually only Einthoven himself and his chief technician had access. With strong illumination however many loose strings subsequently were found floating in the air. The assistants saw little or nothing of this work, partly because strings had to be renewed only rarely (de Waart 1957 [108]). For the mechanically resonant string phonograph dust could not be completely avoided, which affected the definition of the string's image somewhat; de Waart remarks that most dust particles would weigh more than the string itself. Einthoven planned to assemble archives of human speech for analysis. He sent his then chief assistant Hoogerwerf, who in 1924 had written his doctoral thesis on the string phonograph, to Vienna where linguistic records were being filed. However, after Einthoven's death the project was abandoned.

In this last phase of Einthoven's work a specific technical problem (in this case the construction of an extremely thin string and the observation of its deflections) again occasioned scientific investigations in another field. In this particular instance the main question was, how it could be explained that a very thin wire with a diameter in the order of 0.04 μ i.e. equal to or below the diameter of the retinal cones, could be seen separately. The answer proved to be that neighbouring cones of the retina are much more sensitive to differences in light intensity (especially if the string was seen as a shadow against a light background) than to differences in distance between neighbouring objects[50,52]. A problem of a purely physical nature was the Brownian movement of the string in a very high vacuum which was already mentioned.

In his last period Einthoven also found time to write another review of electrocardiography, as he had planned to do for many years (fig.15). It was published posthumously as part of Bethe's "Handbuch für normale und pathologische Physiologie" [61]. Einthoven managed to correct most of the proofs during his final illness, which kept him in hospital for several months. This review is remarkably lucid, more extensive and somewhat easier to read (by avoiding mathematics) than his lecture at the Nobel Prize ceremony a few years earlier [59]. No effort was made however to provide information about recent developments in clinical diagnosis by means of the electrocardiogram such as Einthoven had seen in the U.S.A. While Einthoven maintained his view of the electrocardiogram as an integration of all cardiac potential differences at every single moment, he accepted in fact Lewis' theory of the bicardiogram and the (wrong) terminology of bundlebranch block derived from it; this will be discussed further in chapter 6, section 3.

Einthoven's final illness was caused by abdominal cancer and not connected to his hypertension, of which he had been aware for several years. This hypertension may have been responsible for his recurring attacks of head-ache. On Nov. 22nd 1918 he wrote to Lewis: "I apologize for having waited so long to write to you --- I have repeatedly had head-ache and I fear I am growing old". In 1922 he wrote to one of his daughters: "Yesterday my blood pressure was measured: 240 mM. Furthermore it is only fourteen days ago, that Waller died from a stroke --- It is expected that I shall not last long and that well before my 70th birthday I shall be either seriously ill and invalid or dead ---. (Translation H.A.S.; 70 years was the age of retirement).

Figure 16 (opposite page) *Grave of Willem Einthoven, his wife and his son's ashes; on both sides of it the graves of Mrs Einthoven's relatives (including Willem Thomas de Vogel, the first to publish electrocardiograms from Einthoven's laboratory). At the back the Green Church (so named because of its excessive growth of ivy, now removed). It was built on the site of a wooden chapel reputed to have been consecrated by St.Willibrord in the 8th century. In the 11th century the (tuff stone) church was built, subsequently destroyed in the war against Spain and rebuilt in the 17th century on the old foundations.*

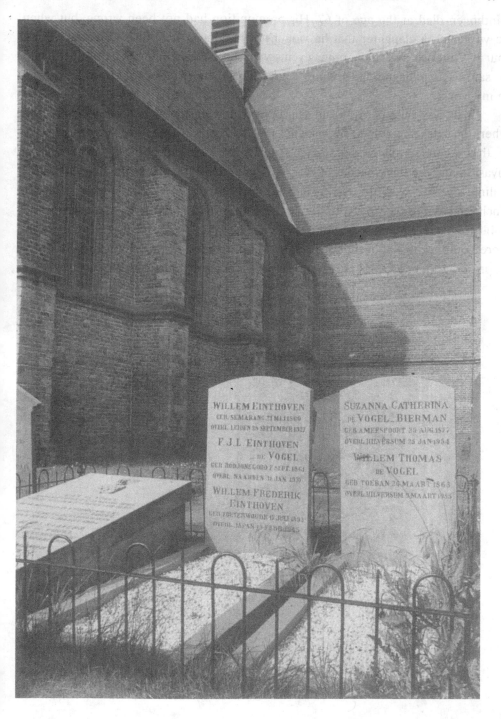

Einthoven died at the age of 67. His premonition had not been wrong, but when he wrote to his daughter that he would not last long, the Nobel Prize,the lecture tour in America and many other events were still ahead. Shortly before his death he said to a colleague and friend: "I have always been in luck, both at home and in my work".

He was buried in an old churchyard at Oegstgeest near Leiden (fig.16), where he later was joined by his wife and the ashes of his son who was director of the radiotelegraphic laboratory of the Dutch East Indies during the Japanese invasion and died as prisoner of war in Japan. This grave is surrounded by a low railing together with the two neighbouring graves of Mrs Einthoven's relatives (including W.Th. de Vogel, Einthoven's brother-in-law and first staff member to publish human electrocardiograms). When it became known, that the three graves were going to be removed, the Einthoven Foundation acquired all three in order to preserve them as a sober memorial to the father of electrocardiography.

Chapter five.

Willem Einthoven and his relatives, friends and personally acquainted scientists.
Part I: Selected Dutch correspondence: Donders, Bosscha, Lorentz, Julius, Wenckebach, de Vogel, W.F. Einthoven, de Waart.

In the foregoing chapters I have tried to picture Einthoven's life and work as far as documented, particularly in the two Dutch biographies by former co-workers mentioned in the Introduction[73,108], Einthoven's own writings and a small selection from his archive, such as two letters to his brother Johan. This chapter will deal with some other Dutch correspondents of Einthoven to wit: one of his teachers (Donders), three physicists (Bosscha, Lorentz, Julius, the last one also being an old friend and brother-in-law), furthermore his fellow medical student and later famous cardiologist Wenckebach, and finally three former co-workers in the laboratory, two of whom had special links with Einthoven, namely his brother-in-law de Vogel, and his son Willem Frederik Einthoven. The latter was not a formal assistant but worked together with his father on the development of the string galvanometer and its use as a receiver of radiotelegrams. The third of the co-workers I shall discuss is de Waart who later became Einthoven's most important biographer.

The appropriate way to arrange this chapter appears to be: writing a series of 8 sections, each covering a brief characterization of one of the correspondents mentioned above and of their respective letters together with their published evaluations of Willem Einthoven. So this chapter (and the following, which deals with selected English and German correspondence) will in fact consist of a series of short sketches with quotations, which together should provide additional information about Einthoven's personality and work by illumination from different angles.

Section 1. F.C. Donders, (1818-1889) was professor at Utrecht University since 1847, initially as extracurricular ("à la suite") professor, who lectured in many subjects but in fact functioned as an unofficial second professor of physiology, specializing in the field of optics. [a] In the latter context he also joined

---

[a] Donders' senior colleague Schroeder van der Kolk combined physiology, anatomy, pathology and psychiatry until his death in 1860.

Bowman of London and von Gräfe of Berlin, as pioneer of clinical ophthalmology; those two became his great friends. He founded the first Dutch Eye Hospital (at Utrecht).

To characterize Donders I can appeal to Einthoven himself, who devoted his first regular lecture to the students after Donders had died, to a commemoration of his revered master. He kept the notes which he made for that purpose. Einthoven praised "his bright intellect and his extraordinary energy, two aspects which always must cooperate". About Donders' lectures Einthoven said: "His lectures were comparable to a beautiful play or opera, of which you don't forget the plot. Donders did not only speak in his lecture, he acted". It was often said that Donders was Einthoven's lifelong example, to whom he frequently referred.[b]

There is little correspondence however. Most of it dates from Donders' last period [c] when his life, already clouded by the death of his daughter in childbed (she was married to Engelmann, Donders' collaborator and successor), became tragic after the prolonged illness and death of his wife and his own increasing disability which he successfully tried to hide. He managed to work on till the glorious formal end of his career in 1888, but died the next year. It is understandable that in the hardly admitted downhill course of his life Donders sought support from his former pupil, now colleague and friend at Leiden. It also quite fitted Einthoven's personality to respond wholeheartedly, for instance by his presence in 1886 at the international meeting of ophthalmologists at Bonn, where Donders handed over the medal commemorating von Gräfe who had already died, to Helmholtz with one of his celebrated speeches.

Section 2. J. Bosscha (1831-1911). Some influential advisers and friends of Einthoven were physicists. The oldest of them was Bosscha, who came into Einthoven's life at a later stage than Donders. After his doctoral thesis in 1854 at Leiden, Bosscha stayed there a few years more as assistant to the physical

---

[b] A statement which Donders made in varying contexts, concerned the value of new methods of investigation. (It was not quoted by Einthoven himself anywhere in his archive, but by de Vogel in his letter to Einthoven of June 19th, 1904 thanking for a reprint of Einthoven's first paper on the string galvanometer): "It is very difficult to make new discoveries along trodden paths.The most important progress in science is brought about by finding new methods of investigation and applying them to old problems, which then can show new aspects and provide unexpected findings".

[c] The only exception occurred when Einthoven was still a medical student. Donders wrote to Einthoven praising his first research (on the movement of the elbow, see chapter 1).

cabinet, went from there to the Military Academy at Breda as professor of physics, then became inspector of education at high schools and subsequently teacher of physics at the polytechnical school of Delft and director of that school (which later rose to University rank and used its new status to give Bosscha an honorary degree). Finally he ended up in 1885 as secretary of the Dutch Society of Sciences at Haarlem. The last function entailed two important tasks: a) that of Curator of Teyler's Museum, one of the oldest (18th century) museums of science and art in the Netherlands and the first to be built expressly for that purpose and b) editor of the Archives Néerlandaises des Sciences Exactes et Naturelles, a Dutch scientific journal in French language.

At the end of the 19th and the beginning of the 20th century, French still was the leading language in diplomatic as well as scientific circles, although on its way to being replaced in the latter context by German and subsequently by English, especially after the second World War. Einthoven repeatedly published in French in Bosscha's journal, but more often in German (Pflügers Archiv der gesamte Physiologie) and occasionally in English [d]. Quite often he published the same or a slightly altered text in more than one foreign language; nearly always preceded by the same paper in Dutch. According to custom his reports to the Royal Dutch Academy were published at the same time in Dutch and in English.

Einthoven's acquaintance with Bosscha through the latter's editorship grew to real friendship; especially after Einthoven published his recently constructed string galvanometer in the issue, which served as Bosscha's "Festschrift" when the latter reached the age of 70. Apart from appreciating the honour, Bosscha was and always remained really intrigued by the string galvanometer and full of admiration for this instrument. For its benefit he devised a plan, whereby Einthoven could obtain a grant of fl. 500 for physiological research from the Society at Haarlem. In this connection Bosscha thought of using the string galvanometer for the reception of the very recently introduced radiotelegraphy

---

[d] Einthoven was reported to have a special gift for languages. This may well be so, but apart from having learned the usual three foreign languages at high school, here again Einthoven did not spare any effort to avoid errors. For the French text in Bosscha's journal there was a regular translator, for the papers in English Waller and Lewis took care of editing the papers published in their respective journals and for German the correspondence shows that Einthoven tried to find a translator; it is not clear, if and how he succeeded in this. Moreover he arranged for lessons in French conversation at supper for a while (in absence of the children) and took English books to bed for reading before dozing off.

and also of enhancing its sensitivity by placing it into a vacuum. Both projects were pondered over by Einthoven but not carried out until his own son came up with the same propositions more than 10 years later.

At this particular moment (1904) Einthoven preferred to use the money for connecting the academic hospital with the physiological laboratory by telephone cable (a telephone system was being installed at Leiden just then by a private firm) in order to make it possible that electrocardiograms were taken from patients. This course of events has been described differently in the literature, even by Einthoven himself who ascribed the initiative to this connecting cable to Bosscha and Professor Place; the latter was president of the Haarlem Society which accorded Einthoven a subsidy. Both correspondence and Einthoven's publications clarify the true state of affairs.

When Bosscha began to think about his retirement, the timing of which he could decide himself, he tried to find a successor whose reputation and scientific standing would ensure the survival of the unique institution which Bosscha was going to leave behind. From his letter to Einthoven of Nov. 16, 1908 it is clear that he approached two professors of physics at Leiden, Lorentz and Kamerlingh Onnes (both Nobel Prize winners but in different years) and a few others without success. However when the succession became urgent after Bosscha died in 1911, an arrangement was made by which Lorentz could continue as part-time professor at Leiden while succeeding Bosscha in a somewhat modified position, in particular through reorganization of the journal. The latter changed its name into Archives Néerlandaises de Physiologie and came under a different editorship.

Section 3. <u>H.A. Lorentz</u> (1853-1928) became a friend and important adviser to Einthoven, who could turn to the former with questions about difficult physical problems. Einthoven probably regarded him as his teacher in a sense, because it was from Lorentz's book that Einthoven learned integral and differential calculus during his first years at Leiden. Or rather, Einthoven saw Lorentz at the same time as a respected master and as an equivalent colleague, but already famous and 7 years older. Einthoven was grateful for advice but even when it came from Lorentz he felt compelled to form and follow his own considered judgement. In his letter of July 24, 1900 Einthoven thanked Lorentz for giving his opinion on one of his papers for Pflüger's Archiv but added that he could not yet decide to embody Lorentz' remarks in his own paper before he had absorbed them fully. So he asked the publisher for permission to wait a few weeks before returning the proofs. In the meantime he could perhaps formulate some further questions. This deferral of decision till all aspects had become clear or confirmed, returns several times at different stages of Einthoven's career.

From several short letters which refer to previous visits or attempts to do so (by the way, never to telephone calls; this means of communication was probably absent in private homes in that first period), it is evident that a true friendship was growing in the course of the years which did not change when Lorentz moved to Haarlem in 1912.

After the first World War there was a new source of rapprochement, because Lorentz then became an important neutral mediator as far as science was concerned, between the victorious and the losing parties. During the last years of the war, as the correspondence shows, Einthoven while approving the denunciation by Lorentz of the brutal horrors of war and his condemnation of the Germans for a broken pledge when they transported Belgian unemployed to Germany, did not sign a letter of protest to the Reichskanzler as Lorentz proposed. It may sound curious - and in the light of our own experience in World War II unbelievably naïve - that Einthoven summed up his objections as a) that war is horrible but that both sides participated in cruelty and unfairness [e], b) that the jobless should themselves prefer useful work to financial support where and whenever work is available. With full approval on the other hand, Einthoven accepted a few years later a suggestion from Lorentz who was from the beginning a member and later president of the "Conseil international de recherches", to support the endeavours of the Dutch Academy of Sciences in favour of admittance of some German scientists to the Conseil (none were invited at its foundation). Lorentz' proposition called for an appeal by a group of Nobel Prize winners who were willing to guarantee the individual admissibility of a number of German scientists (letter of June 24, 1925).

Especially in the letters of this last period Lorentz' personal concern and friendly interest became apparent. For instance: in his letter of congratulation with the Nobel Prize (Nov. 21, 1924) Lorentz remarks that this "recognition of ingenuity and perseverance --- is the more striking, because you always worked in perfect simplicity and modesty". It is also clear how well Lorentz understood and valued Einthoven's affinity with physical principles and methods in applying them

---

[e]   It is possible that this statement had something to do with anti-British sentiments which the war against the Boers in South Africa (Dutch descendants after all) had evoked in many Dutchmen, among them Einthoven.

to physiology (letter of congratulation with Einthoven's doctorate honoris causa in physics at Utrecht in 1913). At the death of Julius (1925) whom Lorentz knew rather well, he tried to visit Einthoven but not finding him, sent a letter of condolence with memories of the deceased whom he described as an "astute researcher and a true-hearted, noble man". On this same occasion Lorentz expressed his concern because Einthoven felt tired after the American tour and the subsequent meeting of the English Physiological Society at Leiden, urging him to "take your ease, which you are fully entitled to".

Section 4. W.H. Julius (1860-1925) was of the same age as Einthoven and an old friend from the time they studied together at Utrecht. Later he married Einthoven's youngest sister. He was still on the staff of the Utrecht Physical Laboratory, when Einthoven (professor at Leiden for 3 years) in 1889 wrote to Julius after receiving the latter's treatise, which had earned him a gold medal. Einthoven congratulated Julius with his success and added that he himself felt very small, looking at Julius' great efforts and excellent results: "How much do I hope that you will soon find a suitable post, where you can work according to your heart's desire, free from worries about your livelihood. Did you send a copy of your book to the professors of physics at Leiden? Don't forget van der Waals at Amsterdam". Another 3 years later Julius was called to Amsterdam as extraordinary professor of physics and in 1896 he returned to Utrecht as full professor of physics, physical geology and meteorology [f].

Einthoven wrote to Julius for advice in physical problems and entrusted him with his plans and difficulties. For instance, in November 1896 Einthoven wanted to talk to Julius and another old friend about the different aspects of Einthoven's intention of asking the university to relieve him from his lectures on histology and physiological chemistry. This matter was already mentioned in chapter 2. On his side Julius when ready to leave Amsterdam, asked Einthoven to come and help him prepare the guidelines for his inaugural address at Utrecht. From then on rather little correspondence is available (and chiefly on family matters) with Julius himself and sometimes with either Einthoven's youngest sister (Mrs Julius) or Einthoven's mother who spent several years of her life with the family at Utrecht.

---

[f]   The latter subject reflects the fact that Julius' predecessor (Buys Ballot) was a pioneer of meteorology. Julius himself became interested in physics of the sun and thereby in astronomy. To the latter discipline a special chair was dedicated after Julius' death.

Most of the correspondence with Julius on scientific and technical matters deals with the characteristics of the capillary electrometer and the necessary correction of its records. The available correspondence covers the period from January, 1894 through June, 1898. It is incomplete on Einthoven's side however, in that copies of Einthoven's letters are lacking until November 1896.

Einthoven and Julius succeeded in arranging the publication in the same issue of Annalen der Physik und Chemie (Nov. 1895) of two papers dealing with their respective methods for the protection of sensitive instruments against mechanical disturbance. In Einthoven's case this concerned the capillary electrometer (see chapter 2). In a letter of 1896, of which no copy has been found, Einthoven asked advice about his endeavours (already mentioned in chapter 2) to realize the design of a secondary ship's compass in the wheel-house steered by the main compass elsewhere in the ship so as to avoid undue magnetic influence by neighbouring steel masses. The idea was welcomed by Julius with interest and admiration. To Einthoven it probably was first of all a scheme by which he hoped to improve his financial situation in his early years at Leiden. Einthoven was no more successful in this than in later projects which could have been profitable. When finally his dual compass system was installed in a ship of the Dutch Navy, his recompensation was no more than a few hundred guilders after deduction of expenses. Einthoven's first thought was about how much of the money should be given to Julius. To a long letter in which Einthoven tried to sort this out in all fairness, Julius replied that the idea was entirely Einthoven's own and that he had been able to help only a little. Therefore he did not want to claim any part of the ridiculously low sum Einthoven had received. If the latter insisted on reimbursing his expenses, then Julius thought that for a return train fare to Leiden from Amsterdam and the loss of an umbrella on that occasion, fl. 25 would be sufficient compensation. The decision about sharing future profits was postponed by Einthoven until other compasses would be sold; there is no record of such an occurrence.

Section 5. K.F. Wenckebach (1864-1941) was a fellow student at Utrecht like Julius, but 4 years younger and studying medicine. He had no influence on Einthoven's career nor was he ever an intimate friend, but in the history of cardiology both Einthoven and Wenckebach became important pioneers, although in a different way. Also in different positions: Einthoven went from Utrecht to the Laboratory of Physiology at Leiden where he remained for the rest of his life, whereas Wenckebach who originally wanted to do histological studies but was prevented by color blindness to do so, worked during his student years with Engelmann in the physiological laboratory. Thereafter he was a general physician at Heerlen and later at Utrecht, all the time studying cardiac arrhythmias in his patients and showing the agreement of his findings with Engelmann's animal experiments. Without any further training Wenckebach became professor of internal medicine at Groningen, Strassbourg and Vienna. Especially at Groningen and Vienna Wenckebach demonstrated also his social qualities as an organizer: At Groningen he was co-founder of the symphony orchestra; at Vienna he promoted a suitable accommodation for the department of medical history in the Josephinum (former military school) and after World War I he asked his many friends abroad to help organize an international food transport (including from former foes) to hunger-stricken Austria. Like Mackenzie he studied external pulsations (venous in the neck, arterial at the wrist and cardiac at the chest wall; especially the last two). Only rather late in his career Wenckebach was won over to electrocardiography.

Perhaps his lack of intimacy with Einthoven had something to do with the fact that the latter could not approve of the methods Wenckebach used, especially the mechanocardiogram (the third method mentioned above). For a physically minded physiologist like Einthoven it was horrifying that the shape of the mechanical cardiogram was so variable and dependent on the positioning of the receiver on the chest, that some investigators only admitted tracings of a predetermined type as reliable. On his side Wenckebach found the external cardiogram as well as the venous and arterial pulse efficient for the timing of the heart beat which was his particular concern. More than once Wenckebach asked Einthoven in one of the few existing letters if he had changed his mind in this respect. The first time Wenckebach did so was connected with Einthoven's paper with Geluk (1894) [23] in which the time relations of mechanogram, phonocardiogram and electrocardiogram as indicators of cardiac contraction were compared. Einthoven's rejection of the shape of the mechanical tracings became outspoken in his paper on "Weiteres über das Elektrokardiogram" of 1908 [35]. (More about the electrocardiogram). In the introduction of this paper Einthoven discussed the mechanocardiogram, the graphic registration of intraventricular pressure - also sometimes called cardiogram - and the E.C.G. from which only the latter two lent themselves to quantitative analysis. It must be remarked, that Einthoven's preference for exact measurements revealed itself also in a negative way, that is in the rather uncharacteristic shape of his pulse and heartbeat tracings to which Einthoven apparently did not pay much attention.

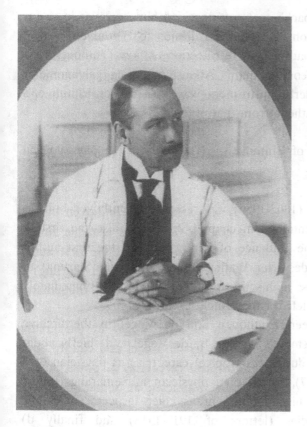

Figure 17. *K.F. Wenckenbach at Vienna in his fifties.*

Instead Einthoven recommended the electrocardiogram as a perfect tool to study arrhythmias. Presumably Wenckebach was disappointed by Einthoven's lack of interest in his clinical studies. In 1914 Einthoven sent congratulations to Wenckebach with his nomination to the chair of medicine at Vienna, but again did not budge concerning the unreliability of the mechanocardiogram. In 1926 Wenckebach inquired if it was true that Einthoven had made a new type of string galvanometer and where one could get it, indicating that he had just finished with Winterberg a book full of electrocardiograms (i.e. Wenckebach's famous book on irregular heart action, published by W. Engelmann, Leipzig 1927) . Einthoven replied that he was glad to hear that and gave the required address.

It appears evident that there was no close friendship between the two such as Wenckebach had with Mackenzie before World War I (however, seeing each other again after the war was a disappointment according to Mair [91]).

Einthoven and Wenckebach may have been too different in several respects. Not only in their career and scientific approach, but also in character: for instance, Wenckebach was much more extravert and assertive, at least in the 1930's when I met him more than once, than Einthoven presumably ever was (fig.17). On the other hand, in his obituary of Einthoven [117] Wenckebach showed to have had a great respect for Einthoven's work since the time that they both studied at Utrecht. On two occasions Einthoven then showed by his own investigations where his teachers had gone wrong and this was readily accepted by both

of them (see chapter 1). Wenckebach's memory deceived him however in so far
as he ascribed Donders' explanation of the optical illusion to Einthoven, who in
fact refuted it. But Wenckebach had a vivid recollection of how Einthoven as a
student was recognized as "the coming man". About the string galvanometer
Wenckebach said that "this wonderful instrument was born out of Einthoven's
head fully developed like Pallas Athene from that of Zeus".

Lastly I include a small selection of Einthoven's co-workers in the physiological
laboratory.

Section 6. W.Th. de Vogel (1863-1955) was related to Einthoven both as
brother-in-law and cousin. As mentioned in chapter 2, he was also the first to
take his doctor's degree under the guidance of Einthoven and the first author
from Leiden (the third world-wide, after Waller and Bayliss with Starling) to
publish human electrocardiograms: in his thesis of early 1893 [107]. Immediately
after finishing his thesis de Vogel left for the Dutch East Indies.

The correspondence between Einthoven and de Vogel in the archive
consists of four groups of letters, mainly written by de Vogel and chiefly about
difficulties which he experienced during his tropical career: a) as physician of a
plantation (letters from 1893-1897), b) as town physician at Semarang (letters
from April-Sept. 1904), c) after his appointment as chief inspector of public
health in the Dutch East Indies (letters of 1917-1918) and finally d)
correspondence in the period that de Vogel lived in Switzerland during a sabbatical year; this period was then prolonged in the context of a special mission of
contact with Europe.

a) In his letter of Dec.10, 1893 de Vogel described his difficulties in the
treatment of his administrative boss for a bone fracture and his own somewhat
neurasthenic uncertainties about it. Also mentioned were his attempts to increase
his income as medical officer in other plantations. In October and November
1897 de Vogel reported to Einthoven about his clinical and experimental studies
of ophthalmology at Heidelberg, during an European furlough.

b) When de Vogel had been town physician at Semarang for a few years,
an order was issued by the Minister of Colonial Affairs which made private
practice impossible for public health officers, whereby his income was reduced
considerably. Thereupon de Vogel asked Einthoven to seek advice in Holland
from former physicians in the Dutch East Indies and to go to the Colonial
Ministry. When Einthoven arrived there, the Minister was absent and Einthoven

was referred from one official to another. All of them proved to be irritated because de Vogel had sent a letter to the Ministry, in which he wanted an answer within half a year, moreover reminding the department of his request by asking well-connected people to intervene on his behalf. A compromise was finally found in the proposal that public health officers in the Dutch East Indies could retain their private practice only in a specialized field. In de Vogel's case this would be ophthalmology. Before this compromise was reached, Einthoven wrote to de Vogel confidentially that the University considered building a new physiological laboratory, which would entail increase of staff and therefore an opportunity for de Vogel to return to Leiden. There is no other record in the Einthoven archive about these plans, nor is it known why they were not realized. Possibly there is a relation with the roofing of the inner court of the laboratory which had been effectuated only a few years earlier and/or the first plans (which would take many years to complete and still more to realize) of transferring the university hospital and the laboratories of anatomy, physiology, pharmacology and pathology together to a common location outside the centre of the town. In any case much later, more or less coinciding with Einthoven's Nobel Prize, an offer to build a new laboratory was received[g] and refused by Einthoven because he could not afford the time for its planning (de Waart [108] and oral reports).

c) In 1917 there was a period of correspondence which this time started with a letter from Einthoven to de Vogel, written at the request of the Leiden medical faculty. De Vogel had become chief inspector of the public health service in the Dutch East Indies and in that quality was adviser on medical matters to the Minister of Colonies. The latter wanted to concentrate the special training for tropical health service in one university instead of the two (Leiden and Amsterdam) which had been functioning so far. In spite of his ties with Einthoven and the University of Leiden de Vogel advised the Minister to prefer Amsterdam and the Minister acted accordingly.

The reason for de Vogel's attitude which he explained both formally to the Leiden faculty, and more extensively in a personal letter to Einthoven revealed de Vogel as an early pioneer of prevention, especially in the situation of a large population, spread out over a cluster of islands as was the case in the Dutch East Indies. At Amsterdam several former members of the medical health service in the Dutch East Indies held positions in the medical faculty, moreover a

---

[g] Fahr [67] described these events as closely related and mentioned even an intervention by the Queen of Holland on this occasion.

Tropical Institute had been installed; preventive measures were taught and propagated there better than at Leiden. On the other hand de Vogel thought it feasible to leave the training of medical officers for the tropical army at Leiden, because for this group the knowledge of individual diagnosis and treatment was chiefly required.

d) After a long letter from de Vogel about a fact-finding visit to the Philippines in 1920, the next group of letters starts with another one from de Vogel who was then in Switzerland for another European year, chiefly because of his wife's health. However, in June 1924 he found himself infected with dysentery of an unspecified character and he did not find any clinician in Switzerland with tropical experience, able to provide adequate diagnosis and treatment. Einthoven sent the information he could get from expert colleagues and offered to come and escort him to Holland but in the meantime de Vogel had been able to obtain the exact diagnosis (amoebic dysentery) and right drug (Yatren - which he had to order in Germany - and emetin) himself. The last letter of this correspondence dates from March 20, 1925 and announces de Vogel's restored health and his decision not to write anymore for fear of taking too much time of Einthoven's busy life.

De Vogel was going to remain in Switzerland because he had been asked to stay in the tropical health service as a liaison officer of the Dutch East Indies with the Ministry of Colonial affairs and the most important international agencies such as the League of Nations and the international office of public hygiene in Geneva. De Vogel survived Einthoven for almost 28 years; he returned to Holland where he died and was buried in the family plot next to Einthoven (see chapter 4 and fig.16).

As far as the character of the correspondence is concerned I should mention that Einthoven and de Vogel, who both had Willem ("Wim" for short) as first name, started many of their letters by addressing each other as "Boy" and "Old one" respectively, although Einthoven was only three years older. In some respects Einthoven's correspondence with de Vogel resembles that with Samojloff, but the latter continued to occupy himself with electrocardiography in contrast to de Vogel. In both cases most of the letters are written to Einthoven, not by him; both correspondents also felt a need of friendship and help at special moments of their lives. Einthoven's reaction was often somewhat reserved, presumably in order to avoid overburdening with information and appeals; on the other hand, if there were serious difficulties he was immediately ready to help.

Section 7. Willem Einthoven's son <u>Willem Frederik Einthoven</u> (1893-1945) was not a formal member of the physiological team nor a physician or a student of medicine; he studied electrical engineering at the Polytechnical College at Delft. However, already during his student days he assisted his father in designing more sensitive versions of the string galvanometer (fig.18). In particular, he proposed the construction of a vacuum string galvanometer and to use this instrument for the reception of radiotelegraphic Morse messages from Java, some 12.000 kilometres (more than 7.000 miles) away. This was already discussed in chapter 4, where it was mentioned that Willem Frederik interrupted his studies to try out this radiotelegraphic connection with the Netherlands. In the 2 years that Einthoven Jr remained in the Dutch East Indies for this purpose, a rather frequent correspondence between him and his father developed, of which only some letters by Einthoven Sr are now in the archive of the Boerhaave Museum. They were kept by his widow after Willem Frederik's death as a prisoner of war in Japan and were given to the present author who passed them on to the Museum Boerhaave to be added to the Einthoven archive. It should be mentioned that Willem Frederik after the final success of the radiotechnical enterprise with the vacuum galvanometer described in chapter 4 and the end of his studies followed by his marriage, went back to the Dutch East Indies where he became chief of the radiotelegraphic laboratory and an internationally respected pioneer in radiotelegraphy until the Japanese invasion of 1942. Willem Frederik was then taken prisoner and transported to Japan where he died in 1945.

The available correspondence is limited and one-sided, as mentioned above. Nevertheless it shows Willem Einthoven's (and his wife's) solicitude for their son's well being as well as the father's concern for the success of their common endeavour. Most of the work had to be done in the tropics and more than once Einthoven Sr waited impatiently for news about it. On both sides the letters were numbered, which compensated somewhat their often irregular and delayed delivery. But there was also a discrepancy between father and son in regularity and frequency of letter writing: in the fall of 1919 the father's letter no. 75 announces the receipt of his son's no. 35. Willem Einthoven also heard about his son from his younger brother Emile, who was in the middle of his tropical career of civil service at various places on Java among them Semarang, where Willem and his brothers and sisters were born. As mentioned earlier (chapter 4), Einthoven Sr felt obliged to keep the real purpose of Willem Frederik's mission in the Dutch East Indies a secret, even from Emile.

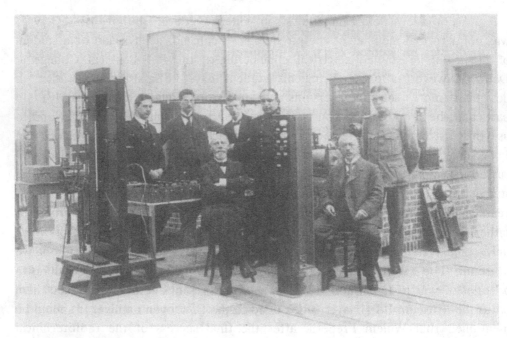

Figure 18 *Scientific co-workers in Einthoven's laboratory during World War 1 (probably 1916 or 1917). Standing from left to right: W.F. Einthoven (son), Hugenholtz (later general physician near Leiden), Waar (later general physician at the Hague), Flohil (later general physician in the east of Holland), Bijtel (later ear specialist at Amsterdam). Sitting: W. Einthoven (left) and Bergansius (physicist). The whole group is gathered around an installation of the string galvanometer (the instrument itself on the pillar behind Einthoven. Left of son Einthoven the standing frame which allows a photographic glass plate to slide down during taking of records (its speed being regulated by a counter weight in oil). In 1933-1935 I worked in the internal department of the Leiden Academic Hospital with such an arrangement (until it was replaced by a much smaller Boulitte model, a fairly recent French construction).*

The available letters show, that father Einthoven studied the vibrations of a cord as model for those of the galvanometer string in particular with relation to waveform and overtones but also to adherent dust particles, represented in the model by pellets of wax. The letters from Einthoven Sr contain some physical and technical advice besides news about the family. Mrs Einthoven mentions her husband's lecture at the Hague, in one of the series of lectures still yearly offered at the concert-hall "Diligentia" near the palace of the Queen Mother who came incognito to listen to him. Apart from Willem Einthoven's paternal and perhaps exaggerated concern for the health of his son, it is evident that Einthoven also worried about his own health. Particularly in connection with the future of his family and more especially of his son who at that moment still had to finish his studies at Delft. After two years father Einthoven asked him to return and to resume his studies while he promised financial support. In relation to the latter Einthoven Sr recalled their agreement that possible profits would be shared; he also made arrangements for an unexpected crisis (e.g. war or his own death).

Section 8. After leaving Leiden A. de Waart (1889-1981) became professor of physiology at the medical school of Batavia (now Djakarta); in 1946 he came back to Leiden as physiologist at the Dutch Institute of Preventive Medicine.[h] There is some correspondence about working again in Einthoven's laboratory in March 1922 during a sabbatical year in order to write a thesis. This did not materialize, chiefly because of difference of opinion on the choice of an investigation that could be done in the available time and its suitability as subject for a thesis. There is also correspondence (or notes on conversation) with him and other assistants (among them Hoogerwerf who substituted after Einthoven's death but was not chosen as successor), about prolonged ties with the laboratory, including possible prospects as lecturer but Einthoven always refused to make promises which he could not be sure to fulfil and repeatedly warned against disappointment.

Three years after de Waart's book on Einthoven was published, a symposium was held in 1960 at Leiden commemorating the centenary of Einthoven's birth. de Waart was asked to speak about Einthoven's personality as

---

[h] Recent inquiries failed to locate de Waart in the register of former staff members of the Institute. Perhaps he was there on a voluntary basis after his retirement from the medical school at Batavia. I used to meet him, while he was working at Leiden, and witnessed his succession by cardiologist Bonjer who for a long time collaborated with the department of cardiology.

a complement to his book of 1957 which mainly deals with Einthoven's work. However, de Waart remarked that in Einthoven's case it is virtually impossible to separate the man and his work; moreover it was contrary to Einthoven's conviction to emphasize his personality [or merits, for that matter]. de Waart's paper was published in the American Heart Journal of March 1961 [109]. I quote:---" In Einthoven's work we notice again and again how he persevered. He could point out to a new assistant on his very first workday the necessity of persevering ---. Besides his will to persevere and his modesty we want to stress his honesty and idealism ---. Einthoven kept his laboratory active and pliable by never trying to build a permanent staff. [i] --- Since most of the experiments could not be carried out without an assistant, the members of the small staff worked as a rule in pairs, each acting as assistant to the other on alternate days ---. Handling the original and for some time the sole galvanometer with its at that time unsurpassed merits was not so difficult. Inserting a new string however, was more complicated and was performed only in the presence of the professor. Yet the same string might last many years ---".

I am ending this section by quoting de Waart's description of Leiden in the early 1900's and Einthoven's life in that town. "During the years I worked with Einthoven, i.e. 1909-1913, Leiden was a very quiet little town. There were hardly any automobiles; at any rate, none of the professors had an automobile. A horse-tram connected the station with de Hogewoerd [that is: from the west to the east city border] ---. Along the Rijnsburgerweg, the narrow road [j] allowing a beautiful view over the meadows as far as the old castle of Poelgeest [k], there was a primitive steam tram. --- This was the favourite road Einthoven chose in the evenings for his stroll. --- Going to his laboratory he always crossed Leiden on bicycle and in case of rain was protected by a very special coat, the kind which was also worn by the celebrated pianist Pembaur. On the last Saturday of each

---

[i]   It can be added that only de Waart himself and the South Africans Jolly and Battaerd remained in physiology and became professor in the Dutch East Indies and in South Africa respectively; all others went into other branches of medicine, in particular general practice or a clinical speciality.

[j]   now the main road from Leiden to the sea-shore.

[k]   Boerhaave lived there for several years during the summermonths and cultivated in its rather large park shrubs and trees for the University's Botanical Garden, of which he was the director.

month, Einthoven could be seen at the station wearing a top hat, on his way to the monthly meetings of the Academy of Sciences".[1]

---

[1] This story is much more likely to be true than Barron's [3] version of Einthoven using his bicycle to cover the distance to Amsterdam (more than 30 miles).

Chapter six.

Willem Einthoven's correspondence with personally acquainted colleagues.
Part II: selected correspondence in English and German:
Fahr, Waller, Lewis, Wilson, Samojloff, A.V. Hill, Wiggers. Review of their papers on Einthoven.

In this chapter some of the correspondence in English and German is discussed together with publications on Einthoven by most of the correspondents. German quotations are given in English translation. We start with George E. Fahr, who in fact represents a transition between chapter 5 ending with co-workers of Einthoven, to whom Fahr belonged and chapter 6 about foreign correspondents and authors of papers on Einthoven, a group he also was part of.

Section 1. George Fahr (1882-1968) studied with M. von Frey at Würzburg when he wrote to Einthoven in 1907 asking if he could come and work with him. He did not mention, that von Frey had recommended to do so and therefore Einthoven, always cautious, first asked von Frey if he knew about it before answering Fahr. The latter came to Leiden for half a year in 1910 on a voluntary basis and subsequently for a year as regular assistant in 1911-1912. Von Frey had already frequently corresponded with Einthoven, mainly requesting photographs or diapositives of Einthoven's tracings which he wanted to use in his own lectures and papers, but once also asking Einthoven to lecture at the German congress of scientists and physicians at Karlsruhe (published in 1912 [41]). Moreover, von Frey inquired after Einthoven's opinion on commercially available string galvanometers. On May 26, 1911 he was answered by Einthoven that a perfect instrument was not yet available at the moment. "In many respects the Cambridge Instrument Company produces a very acceptable galvanometer with an excellent string, but the magnification by its microscope is not optimal".

In 1914 von Frey wrote that he had received a long paper from Fahr on the theory of the string galvanometer for publication in the Zeitschrift für Biologie of which he was editor. He told Einthoven that the paper was mainly theoretical and not aggressive, but that he would not publish it if Einthoven did not approve. Einthoven answered that Fahr had done something similar already in offering a paper to the American Journal of Physiology without Einthoven's knowledge, only informing him afterwards by telephone. Einthoven found this unsympathetic and did not want to read that paper at such a late date. Very likely it was the same paper which was rejected by the American Journal of Physiology probably because of its length, that now had been sent to von Frey in German language. Einthoven decided that his own feelings were not important, only the paper's scientific value, and asked von Frey to judge it accordingly. The latter intended to accept it, but the publication cannot be found in the series of that journal; perhaps because World War I broke out soon afterwards.

This episode is interesting because it reveals Einthoven's attitude in relation to his personal feelings. They never were an obstacle to good relations at a later date; as far as Fahr is concerned it is known that he always admired Einthoven (see below). He helped organize Einthoven's lecture tour in the U.S.A.; at that occasion Einthoven was his guest at Minneapolis.

The correspondence between Einthoven and Fahr is limited and does not offer much information except with relation to the lecture tour. However, when at Fahr's 80th anniversary his friends at Minneapolis, were he had been a professor of internal medicine for many years, published a "Festschrift" for him, he contributed himself to this publication by relating his reminiscences of Einthoven and the latter's laboratory at Leiden under the title: Ik wilde weten [a] (I wanted to know, [67]). This provided an interesting but curious story, that is compounded from true devotion and astute observation and on the other hand some partially or wholly wrong statements, as other sources and Einthoven's own archive and writings reveal. The errors can sometimes be identified as false interpretation of true facts, or distortion of information by failing memory after a long time: at times Fahr's original information may have been incorrect to begin with, even if it came from Einthoven himself (according to Fahr, that is).

For instance: Fahr reports that Einthoven told him that his father was a descendant of Spanish Jews, who had emigrated to Holland hundreds of years before and who married a Dutch woman. On comparing this with the true course of events as described in the first chapter, it will be seen that there are a few correct elements in an otherwise muddled story. It concerns in fact Einthoven's grandfather who died before Willem Einthoven was born. He was the first to assume the name of Einthoven and after a few years in England returned to his

---

[a]   This was Einthoven's answer to inquisitive reporters at the time of his Nobel Prize, when he was asked to tell how his successful research came about..

country as assistant military surgeon by way of Spain and Waterloo. Perhaps Einthoven was not interested to check the accuracy of family tales.

Another example is Fahr's assertion that Einthoven after having received the money of the Nobel Prize spent much time in trying to find out whether his former chief mechanic, who was largely responsible for the construction of the first string galvanometer, was still alive. This is easily disproved by the obituary which Einthoven wrote of his valuable technical helper and chief of workshop van der Woerd in 1915. The second half of this information, i.e. that van der Woerd's two daughters were found in straitened circumstances and that Einthoven gave them half of the prize money, may be correct but is difficult to prove as there are no documents on this matter in the Einthoven archive. They would have been unlikely to be kept by him anyway as they would indicate a generosity, which Einthoven probably would not want to be known. Perhaps there is a faintly suggestive indirect evidence: no mention was ever made, orally or in script, about what Einthoven did with the Nobel prize money, except that on its reception he presented each current member of the technical staff with silver cutlery for one person. This was considered a meagre share of the prize money by some as I know from oral reports, but in fact it may have been a small part of what Einthoven gave to the descendants of his first and most helpful chief technician.

A third, less important, aspect concerns Fahr's - correct - information that Einthoven was a sportsman in his student years and practised fencing besides rowing and athletics. However, having studied in Germany, Fahr supposed that fencing automatically meant duelling and he wondered about the absence of corresponding scars on Einthoven's face. This finding should not have been surprising because duelling never was a tradition among Dutch students, in contrast to Germany. Fahr quoted the book by de Waart on Einthoven of 1957 more than once, but apparently did not notice that de Waart mentioned fencing only as a special form of exercise.

One interesting story concerning Fahr himself was already mentioned: he would have liked to stay on at Leiden as a personal link between the hospital and the physiological laboratory with its precious string galvanometer. In retrospect it is perhaps to be deplored that Fahr's wishes were not fulfilled; good cooperation with an interested clinician would have been profitable. However, conditions and persons involved were prohibitive and while it is possible that electrocardiography could have developed better and faster, it is just as likely that Fahr's interposition might have introduced complications.

In any case, around 1910 or a little later, Einthoven began to rely on the clinical and experimental acumen of Thomas Lewis, while he abstained from statements outside his own experience apart from approval of Lewis' theory of bundlebranch block; see section 3 of this chapter. In 1920 Fahr was more successful than Einthoven in detecting a flaw in Lewis' concept and nomenclature by studying the successive changes in direction of the electrical axis; a statement which Lewis dismissed as irrelevant and Einthoven failed to support.

Section 2. <u>A.D. Waller</u> (1856-1922) was responsible or rather, provided the opportunity for Einthoven's choice of electrocardiography as the main object of his scientific research, but he did not share Einthoven's view of its future importance. A man with many different aspects, controversial, endowed with outspoken friends and enemies (according to the obituary by W.L. Symes [104]), he was the first to demonstrate the human electrocardiogram, but hardly one of the staunch promoters of electrocardiography. Waller was strongly influenced by the example of his father, who was professor of physiology at Paris and a pioneer in neurophysiology. In A.D. Waller's eyes his father A.V. Waller was a discoverer with brilliant ideas, (as enumerated in the dedication of the son's textbook of human physiology, 1891 [112]) but perhaps not or at least not in the first place, a persistent perfectionist in search for the complete truth. A.D. Waller's youth in France and his fluency in French (and German after his study with Ludwig in Leipzig) made him free from British insularity to an exceptional degree.

With the support of his wife, who was his ex-student and lifelong collaborator and with her financial help as well as that from her brothers (their father Sir George Palmer was a wealthy man through the Huntley and Palmer's biscuits) Waller had many opportunities for work at his disposal. He had a completely furnished laboratory at home as well as in St. Mary's Hospital and later London University, all of which were equipped in first instance from private means (e.g. by transferring instruments from his home). Waller's interest was virtually all-round but particularly focused on methods and instruments of investigation with a preference for the simplest types. This made him close to Marey and when the latter finally could realize his International Institute at Paris, Waller became after a while its vice-president.

Waller's relation to Einthoven greatly depended on his interest in and admiration of the latter's inventive skill, but he could not understand let alone match, Einthoven's far-reaching vision of clinical electrocardiography nor the systematic and thoughtful way, in which Einthoven made its development possible. This becomes evident for instance, from Waller's paper of 1909 [113] after a visit to Leiden (in fact not primarily for studying electrocardiography but retinal action currents). He made this clear again in 1913 [114], when he assumed that Einthoven would share his opinion that the rôle of the string galvanometer in clinical diagnosis would remain limited to special cases.

On the other hand, Waller wrote in the same year 1913 [b] in the New York Medical Journal [116] (as summary of his Harvey Lecture there) a paper in which he warned against the already general acceptance of the electrocardiographic signs of ventricular hypertrophy, which he considered not sufficiently proven. At the same time he asked attention for a clinical investigation of his own (unproven and implausible) concept that a vertical position of the heart signifies "cor longum et durum" (long and hard), a more horizontal situation "cor brève et molle" (short and soft) with the clinical implication of strong and weak respectively (instead of a simple explanation like varying height of the diaphragm).[c] The paper ends however with the assertion that the "electrocardiographic apparatus or the oscillometer (around this time Waller sought to replace the string galvanometer by this simpler, in fact older and less sensitive instrument) --- is no longer a laboratory toy --- but it is an instrument of great clinical value ---. A "last appeal" was made for the adoption of a "more rational naming" of the several waves of the electrocardiogram (presumably his own or something like it) as opposed to the generally adopted nomenclature because the latter was meaningless. This however was precisely Einthoven's intention: he wanted to leave room for additional findings and new concepts.

However this may be, Waller subsequently took electrocardiograms of soldiers during World War I and later of patients in the National Heart Hospital but could not or rarely persuade other students of electrocardiography to accept his deviating proposals. Not without reason, as the above short review may have shown.

---

[b]   The same subject was treated more extensively in Waller's Oliver Sharpey Lectures published in The Lancet of 1913 [115]. These lectures are unusually explicit in comparing the leads and terminology of Einthoven (called the "usual ones") to Waller's own, which he continues to prefer (combined with his new concept of "long" and "short" hearts).

[c]   Perhaps the sometimes difficult distinction between horizontal heart and left hypertrophy was of influence here.

The correspondence between Einthoven and Waller is interesting, in particular with regard to their different outlook and way of living, and their often similar choice of research projects, how different their approach to them might be. For understanding the latter point Waller's (and Einthoven's) published papers are more clarifying than their correspondence, but both show a mixture of similar and very divergent characteristics. From 1890 on, that is Waller's first letter to Einthoven, various topics of Einthoven's research, from the optical illusion in Einthoven's doctoral thesis to the psychogalvanic reflex in his last period were picked up by Waller or alternatively, very similar topics were chosen independently and subsequently discussed in correspondence or studied together at Leiden. Or again, Waller encouraged publication of Einthoven's results in English. Waller appears to have had a permanent urge to spread his interest and tackle new problems, while Einthoven's period of wide scientific orientation virtually ended at the turn of the century with his concentration on electrophysiology, especially of the heart.

The correspondence extends from 1890 through 1921, the year before Waller died. There are large gaps however; before 1901 there are only three letters written by Waller in the nineties (2 in 1890, 1 in 1892) and none by Einthoven. (This must be due to the fact that Einthoven did not make copies of his own letters before 1896). From 1901 on, Einthoven's letters to Waller (or Mrs Waller, because she sometimes wrote in his name; these were the only occasions that Einthoven asked his own wife to answer for him) were put down as abstracts in Einthoven's own hand until he apparently felt that his copying technique had become adequate.

The first letters from Waller are concerned with Einthoven's research on the optical illusion of perspective by colour difference and on bronchial constriction in asthma as shown by measurement of intratracheal pressure. In both cases Waller discussed ways to make Einthoven's results better known in the English speaking world of physiologists and clinicians, in particular by publication in Brain, of which Waller was sub-editor, later editor. Einthoven's explanation of the optical illusion interested Waller very much, but in repeating the experiment with slight variations, he noticed that he could experience the same illusion even with one eye shut i.e. without stereoscopy. Here again Einthoven could furnish a satisfactory explanation which he published together with his report on his use of Waller's modification, whereby shadows were introduced (see chapter 2). On the other occasion Waller urged Einthoven to give a name to his arrangement for measuring intrabronchial pressure ("I find myself saying pulmonary rheotome in

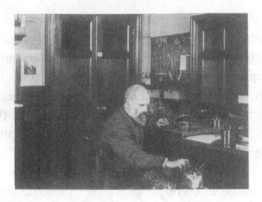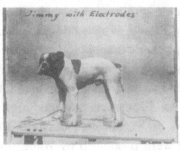

Figure 19.   *A.D. Waller was in his early thirties (here stroking his cat), when he discovered the possibility of recording "the human heart effects". Jimmy was his favorite (and patient) dog for demonstrations.*

lecturing or talking, led to do so perhaps by the expression pulmonary catheter. But you are the father of this child, what will you call it, for give a name you must"). Einthoven apparently did not answer this challenge. In a following letter Waller confirms the receipt of an English text by Einthoven (which subsequently appeared in Brain in 1893 [20]) and asks for a short introductory account of Eintho- ven's earlier paper on the same subject, to avoid misapprehension such as he had encountered recently ("In German or French to be translated. With regard to your English manuscript, it is very good but in places it needs editing").

Reviewing the correspondence in chronological order we must start with a letter of which no copy exists. In 1890 Einthoven apparently had written to Waller that he had made electrocardiograms. At the end of his first letter (Sept 1, 1890) Waller replies: "I am particularly glad to hear that you have been demonstrating the human heart effects, do you find the results as I described them, or do you find any differences? I am sorry I did not receive your letter until after my return from Berlin, I should have been tempted to break the journey at Leiden. However I do not feel Leiden to be very far from London and perhaps you may one day reflect that London is not very far from Leiden" (fig.19).

    In November and December 1903 there is a vivid but somewhat confusing correspondence because Waller wants to come and see the recently published string galvanometer, but likes to combine this trip with a holiday at Berlin or in the surrounding country. Ultimately he writes on Jan. 8, 1904 from the Palace Hotel at St. Moritz in Switzerland (!) where he had arrived for the last week of his holiday. He had also made various plans to take his three children together or separately with him to see Berlin and to let one of his sons stay for a longer period in order to learn German. In the end he visited Leiden with a colleague on his way out and announced from St. Moritz that he would come again with his wife on the way back. Even though Einthoven had let him know that he could not receive him at that date (Jan. 4, 1904), Waller writes from the hotel Lion d'Or at Leiden that he had arranged meeting his wife there and that they would have dinner before sailing to London. Presumably Einthoven did not meet the Waller's at that time; he had invited them for another date to stay in his own home ("if you do not mind to live as simply and plainly as we do").

The correspondence of March 19-22, 1904 centers around a visit to Leiden in the Eastern holidays which Einthoven could not accept [d], because he had to make up for unfinished work due to a previous illness and also concerns the difficulties of Waller to obtain a galvanometer. In the meantime he had received propositions from Duddell (connected with Cambridge Scientific Instruments) to make the instrument in London. However, at that moment Einthoven wrote back that his arrangement with Edelmann as the sole producer had been concluded and the deliverance of either a big model with an electromagnet or a small with permanent magnet would soon be possible. In the next chapter the subsequent difficulties with Edelmann will be discussed, which offered new opportunities to Cambridge Scientific Instruments or Cambridge Instruments Company, as it later was called (see Burnett [9]).

On April 18th 1905 Waller wrote to Einthoven: "I am still languishing for a string galvanometer. I wonder, whether I shall ever have the chance of reproducing the beautiful records you gave me! And I want it for other purposes. May I some day come this summer and use yours?"--- The answer from Einthoven must have been disappointing: "It is really an impossibility for me to give the string galvanometer out of my hands. It is used by myself, my assistants and moreover two pupils who are working at their dissertation. Everybody is busy

---

[d] In a subsequent letter (May 12,1909) Mrs Waller mentioned that they immediately arranged to use the planned week's holiday to sail to Gibraltar and see some parts of southern Spain. This part of the correspondence was conducted between Mrs Waller and Mrs Einthoven.

with it from the morning till the evening, except at the necessary holidays, when the laboratory is shut. I think that we shall not have finished the most pressing work for the first two years. Thereafter it will be a great pleasure to me, to assist you and other physiologists who are inclined to come at Leiden for work with the string galvanometer".

On Dec. 28, 1905 Waller sends a telegram : "Have you skating. Waller". To which Einthoven replied: "Yes Einthoven". A few days later Mrs Waller writes to Mrs Einthoven without referring to the telegram, about her two sons (the older at Berlin learning German, the second preparing for Oxford) and tells that Waller plans to come with his second son to Holland for a few days of skating. It is not known, if Einthoven participated in the skating, although he was fond of it. Perhaps Einthoven saw this plan as another gentle hint with respect to the string galvanometer.

In 1908 publication is discussed of a short account of Einthoven's paper on vagus currents [38] (already published in German [39]) and a new paper by Einthoven and Jolly on action currents of the retina in the Quarterly Journal of Experimental Physiology [37], of which Waller is now editor. Again Waller is very much interested, particularly in the second subject on which he gathers personal experience and tries some modification, such as previous massage of the eyeball. With difficulty a date is agreed in 1909 for Waller and Jolly to come to Leiden and do an experiment together with Einthoven. Beforehand Waller asks for and receives an original negative with some prints and diapositives bearing on the same subject for a lecture he is going to give. From the correspondence one can witness the anxiety of Einthoven as to the return of his negative (and also his modestly expressed insistence on the mention of its origin).

In the following years (1911-1913) there is correspondence with questions from Waller and answers from Einthoven about such divergent topics as the Leiden dissertation by Herbert Mayo in 1818, the calculation of the angle of the electrical axis and the fate of the patient with mitral stenosis in whose E.C.G. Einthoven recognized the pattern of right ventricular hypertrophy. After much trouble Einthoven found out that she died a few months after the electrocardiogram was made; Waller replied that he had a similar case with also an unfavourable clinical course. Apparently he was more inclined to interpret the electrocardiographic pattern as a prognostic sign than as the expression of a functional and/or anatomical change of the heart muscle. In subsequent years Waller repeatedly showed his doubt about empirically found signs of hypertrophy in the E.C.G., now familiar to all cardiologists.

The correspondence then ceased during World War I and was only renewed in 1921 by the demand of Waller for a reprint of Einthoven's paper with de Roos on the electrical aspects of the psychogalvanic reflex [51]. This was a paper published in Dutch and his request for it also was written in - somewhat obsolete - Dutch. The next year Waller died; there is a copy of Einthoven's letter to Mrs Waller ("Waller has had a marked influence on my own scientific work. His famous researches on the electric phenomena of the heart and his beautiful demonstrations at congresses were for me the starting point of a new series of my own investigations. He was a man of world-renown".) Within a year Mrs Waller also died. Her daughter Mary informed Einthoven: "They were only separated for 7 months".

As a summary of Waller's guidelines for his work, A.H. Sykes in 1987 [103] quoted Waller as stating: "my conviction is that while it is essential that scientific inquiry should be pursued for its own sake without regard to its immediate utility, its ultimate justification consists in its practical application to the service of Mankind". To which Sykes adds: "But by this he meant that the physiologist should uncover basic truths in the laboratory which others would then take up and develop in the hospital".

It is interesting to see how close - in spite of many differences of another kind - this view is to Einthoven's own ideas; except however for the two decisive additional steps that required much insight and effort, namely 1) laying a firm quantitative foundation for a controllable and comparable E.C.G. registration everywhere and 2) demonstrating its clinical relevance. This is in fact what Einthoven did. It should be recognized however, that Waller's intuitive approach (largely without actual measurements) sometimes came very near to the truth, at least in the late 1880's when his mind was focused on the action currents of the human heart (see for instance Waller's scheme of potential distribution on the chest of 1889 as compared with much later schemes by others based on results of exact measurements). It was only in the last part of his career (1913-1922) that Waller may have felt so much overshadowed by "Einthoven's electrocardiography", that he opposed some of its concepts and tried to go back to his original own method and ideas of 25 years earlier. It must be added that Waller never attacked Einthoven personally nor mentioned his objections in letters to Einthoven. Waller even virtually never mentioned Einthoven's name in connection with electrocardiography after his report on visiting Leiden in 1909; even while criticizing the "usual" methods of electrocardiography in his Oliver-Sharpey Lectures of 1913 [115], see also footnote *b* of this chapter.

Section 3. <u>Sir Thomas Lewis</u> (1881-1948). In May 1908 Thomas Lewis wrote to Einthoven, his senior by more than 20 years, a respectful letter beginning with "Dear Sir" in which he asked for a reprint of Einthoven's paper "Le Télécardiogramme" [33], the first paper ever about electrocardiograms from patients taken with the new string galvanometer which Einthoven had devised and constructed a few years earlier. Unfortunately Einthoven had no more reprints in stock, but he sent the recently published sequel to that paper, for which Lewis thanked him. The next year however Lewis wrote that he had ordered a string galvanometer from Edelmann and asked about special features. (Another few years later Cambridge Scientific Instruments constructed its own model and gave a galvanometer to Lewis on "loan", which after many years of use was finally bought for a nominal fee). On August 18, 1909 Lewis wrote asking if he could come early in September and see the string galvanometer at work.

This was the beginning of a correspondence of nearly 20 years, interrupted only in the last two years of World War I. Gradually the letters changed their formal beginning to "Dear Professor Einthoven" and finally to "My dear Lewis" and "Dear Einthoven". A true friendship developed, although there always remained a certain distance such as between a beloved pupil and his venerated teacher. The letters were in fact often concerned with questions from Lewis and answers by Einthoven about problems of the former, mostly of a physical nature and related to the instrument, its registration and the interpretation thereof. But at the same time Lewis revealed himself as a deft and inventive experimentalist and a good clinician to boot; for Einthoven the ideal partner in the development and worldwide introduction of electrocardiography. On June 22nd, 1911 Einthoven wrote to Lewis, "An instrument takes its true value not so much from the work it possibly might do, as in fact from the work that it really does".

Thus a mutual affection and respect developed and facilitated a tacit understanding to communicate to each other whatever seemed useful while both retained the freedom of choosing their own field of work without interference by the other. Einthoven always felt grateful for the work done by Lewis, but often was the latter's guide because Lewis was well aware of his own deficient knowledge of physics and mathematics.

However, Einthoven was not the only nor the first friend and guide of Lewis. Before the latter began to use the string galvanometer he made a study of venous tracings and thereby came into contact with Mackenzie, who had recently arrived in London and was already approaching the height of his fame. At that

TO

JAMES MACKENZIE

AND

WILLEM EINTHOVEN

A TOKEN OF APPRECIATION

OF THE SERVICES WHICH THEY HAVE RENDERED

TO THE STUDY OF THE

CLINICAL PATHOLOGY OF HEART AFFECTIONS.

Figure 20. *Dedication of Lewis' book: "The mechanism of the heart beat" (1911) to Mackenzie and Einthoven.*

particular moment Mackenzie was at a loss how to explain the tracings which at first he thought to indicate auricular paralysis because of the absence of atrial waves in the venogram, and later nodal tachycardia. Lewis subsequently identified them as auricular fibrillation (already well known from animal experiments) with the help of the string galvanometer and by following a fibrillating horse to the slaughterhouse, where he could actually see the fibrillating atrium.

Einthoven's letter of June 22nd, 1911 referred to above, was intended to thank Lewis for the latter's book on "The mechanism of the heart beat" [87], which was dedicated to Mackenzie and Einthoven jointly (fig.20). Lewis' friendship with Mackenzie was both more intimate and more ambiguous than with Einthoven (Mackenzie's biographer Mair writes about a love-hate relationship with Lewis). Although Lewis abandoned Mackenzie's method and for several years exclusively studied electrocardiography, Mackenzie was never out of Lewis' thoughts; least of all when the former died in 1925. On Jan. 26, 1925 Lewis wrote to Einthoven: "I would have replied before to your kind letter, but the death of my old friend Mackenzie filled my thoughts".

It seems to me that it is perhaps not a coincidence that at about the same time Lewis turned to quite different subjects of research which in fact were more or less connected with Mackenzie. Of course there may be other reasons which Lewis did not acknowledge publicly nor write about to Einthoven; co-workers mentioned a) weariness of being tied to an instrument (again reminiscent of Mackenzie), b) that "the cream was off" i.e. the subject of electrocardiography was exhausted, which of course proved incorrect. Another, additional reason may have been some disappointment from not having shared Einthoven's Nobel Prize, as was proposed by A.V. Hill (see [102]) and certainly would have been welcomed by Einthoven.

However, Lewis' satisfaction at Einthoven's award (see below) was doubtless genuine. The circulation of the skin increasingly began to draw his attention; he studied dermatographism and made his important discovery of independent contraction of the capillaries almost simultaneously with similar work by Christian Bohr (physiologist and father of the famous physicist Niels Bohr). Lewis' second subject was pain, a favourite topic of Mackenzie in connection with angina pectoris.

Shortly before the end of the Einthoven-Lewis correspondence their only collision almost occurred when Lewis heard from his assistant Craib in the fall of 1926 that he supposed Lewis' theory of limited potentials as put forward in his Mellon's Lecture (1922 [88]) to have emanated from Einthoven. Possessing an archive with copies of his own letters which Lewis did not, Einthoven could show, by sending to Lewis copies of his earlier letters, that he had always considered this as a concept of Lewis; having only added himself the suggestion that the limited spaces where the action potentials supposedly originate, must be the cardiac segments (at that time not yet recognized as cells by histologists, as the myocardium was considered a syncytium).

To set the record straight it is perhaps interesting to point out that Einthoven repeatedly, the first time in 1908 (Weiteres über das E.K.G., [35]) i.e. soon after Tawara's paper on the conducting system [106], but more explicit in 1912 (Über die Deutung des Elektrokardiogramms [42]) asserted that the electrocardiogram at every instant is determined by the summation of all the potential differences in the heart at that moment, irrespective of their location. In the second paper mentioned above (1912), it is made clear that there must be little time difference in the arrival of the excitation wave at corresponding places of the respective surfaces of the right and left ventricle (as beautifully demonstrated subsequently in the dog by Lewis in 1914-'15 [85,86]).

In retrospect we can see therefore that Lewis' concept of "limited" (i.e. sharply localised) potential differences in his Mellon Lecture of 1922 [88] and

Einthoven's suggestion of the myocardial segments (cells) as their location see above, were the logical steps to take after Einthoven's prior notion of multiple, more or less simultaneous but dispersed myocardial excitations.[e]

In a sense Einthoven can be said to have helped paving the way for the concept of cellular myocardial physiology. In "Über die Deutung" [42] mentioned above, Einthoven spelled out the existence of various old and new theories about myocardial contraction and their relation to action current. He concluded that progression of a wave of excitation was the most accepted notion, which however could be linked with more than one theory. But Einthoven never made a choice between existing theories; neither did he create a new one. Presumably he did not expect in the immediate future a new and effective method of exploring the unknown but in his opinion surely existing biochemical processes inside the myocardial microscopical segments (= cells). In any case Einthoven, for many years a teacher but not an investigator of histology, clearly suspected a greater independence of the myocardial cells than was accepted by common opinion.

There are other interesting sidelights in the correspondence: for instance, when Lewis asked why Einthoven had chosen the scheme of an equilateral triangle to define the electrical axis ("--- in the dog it is much more nearly a right angled triangle. I have been puzzled to know whether the adoption of the equilateral triangle introduces any material error in the calculation of the electrical axis ---"), Einthoven replied on Feb. 5, 1915 that he had tried several triangles for his calculations. But: "the most practical one is the equilateral triangle. As soon as we take an other form we shall meet with more difficulties ---". After enumerating the difficulties in the rectangular and isosceles [f] triangles Einthoven concluded: "With the equilateral triangle none of those questions arise --- On the other hand the calculation of the axis in the equilateral triangle is easy".

"Moreover I think that you will not make an error of any practical value if you take the equilateral triangle for the dog as well as for man. I am sorry that my own work on the subject has had to be delayed and I am anxious to see the

---

[e] In his letter of Nov 12, 1926 to Craib in order to set Lewis' mind at rest (see above) Einthoven wrote: "Your remarkable work corroborates and extends the work of Lewis and at the same time it supports my theory of the contracting muscle segments constituting separate electrical units".

[f] with two symmetrical legs.

results that you may obtain--- "(see my editions of the Einthoven-Lewis correspondence [102] and of Einthoven's selected papers. [101])

Lewis thanked Einthoven for his comments adding: "I fear that I have
insufficient knowledge of trigonometry, fully to appreciate your explanation; so I
propose relying upon your conclusion that the equilateral triangle is the most
satisfactory". Prior to this (i.e. October-November 1913), the calculation of the
direction (angle) of the electrical axis had also been a subject of discussion.
Lewis felt uncertain because of a paper by Waller. ("I see that Waller wishes to
explain the curves of hypertrophied hearts on the basis of a displaced axis"; see
also end of section 2 of this chapter). From a series of electrocardiograms of left
and right hypertrophy Lewis then took the mean values of height for R and T,
which seemed to contradict Waller's conclusion. Einthoven answered that Lewis'
calculations were not good and invited him to come to Leiden for the weekend,
and bring many of his tracings. Lewis did not see a possibility to leave London,
so Einthoven tried to explain by letter and announced his plans to write another
paper on the calculation of the axis (not giving particulars). On Nov. 13th, 1913
Lewis answered that he now understands his error "It is very obvious to me now
that you have explained it, and I see that I must calculate the angle for each case
separately. I look forward with pleasure to your further communication. I am
sure I shall profit by it. I hope you will not forget that we shall be only too glad
to take any paper of yours which you propose to publish in Heart ---."

It is not clear which subsequent paper was meant by Einthoven. The same
question had been treated in the Lancet of 1912 [43] and more fully in Pflüger's
Archiv of 1913 [46]. Both of these papers were known to Lewis; so it is likely that
Einthoven planned a third paper, but never got around to it. Probably the
publication of Flohil's dissertation on the relation of electrical and fluoroscopic
(i.e. anatomical) heart axis (see chapter 4) in 1928 [68], a year after Einthoven's
death, must be taken as an indication of Einthoven's unfinished work on this
topic. Flohil's main conclusion, already mentioned, was that anatomical and
electrical axis are not the same, but that changes in direction occur simultaneously and are more or less equal.

It may be pointed out, that Einthoven as a rule limited himself to the
physical and mathematical aspects and left out (not entirely, if one reads his
papers carefully) clinical and related physiological aspects of e.g. left ventricular
hypertrophy and left axis deviation which he probably felt to be in Lewis'
territory of study.

From other topics on the interface of their respective fields of interest I shall mention one more, because it shows the consequences of a more readily accepting attitude on the part of Einthoven. One of the main concerns of Lewis always was to deduce the pathway of the spreading excitation in the heart from the shape of the electrocardiogram. Lewis at first tried to follow Waller and others in tracing the path of excitation spread in terms of direction from base towards apex or vice versa. At this point Einthoven was adamant in asserting that there was no criterion to recognize the pathway of excitation from the shape of the QRS complex; more than once he pointed out that we only can be sure that at every instant the ECG reflects the sum total of all local electrical activities of the heart. About ten years after the anatomy of the conduction system as a whole had became clear from Tawara's paper of 1906 [106]; Lewis himself contributed greatly to the knowledge of the arrival time of excitation impulses especially on the epicardium, which depends on their propagation in either specific conduction tissue or heart muscle and the respective velocities of conduction.

Subsequently Lewis felt the need however to consider the two ventricles as separate but normally strictly cooperating parts of the myocardium, the harmonization of which could be disrupted by disease or experimental cutting of one of the two bundlebranches. This view seemed established at the time by Rothberger and other investigators in Vienna both experimentally and pathologically, and appeared to be confirmed by Lewis and the work of his associates. In retrospect the validity and in particular the completeness of their findings is in doubt as well as the equalization of the experimental and the clinico-pathological data. [8] I do not propose to go into details here; some were mentioned in my publication of the complete correspondence between Einthoven and Lewis [102] and a more extensive review was given by Hollman in his paper "History of bundle-branch block". [72]

From several points of view this episode is interesting: first of all, because the concept of Lewis of the electrocardiogram as a bicardiogram (left + right) led to a wrong conclusion regarding the anatomic and functional localization of bundlebranch block in man among virtually all cardiologists during 20 years or so. This included Einthoven, who refrained from critically examining the founda-

---

[8] Nor was the normally existing difference in thickness of the left and right ventricular myocardium (related to the difference in aortic and pulmonary blood pressure) taken into account. Moreover, disease of a bundlebranch is seldom if ever, strictly limited to one branch. This point was missed because the microscopic examination of serial sections was incomplete.

tions of Lewis' pet theory although fully maintaining his principle, that the E.C.G. is produced by all active parts of the myocardium together, irrespective of how they are grouped anatomically. He was impressed by the (seemingly) conclusive and consistent concept of Lewis, based on anatomical and experimental findings. In addition, Einthoven himself contributed a perhaps deceptive support of Lewis' theory when he showed in a patient whose sternum had been removed, that mechanical stimulation of the (supposedly) right ventricle produced an extrasystole of the dextrogram type [59]. The underlying assumption that right ventricular extrasystoles must always show the same pattern irrespective of their region of origin, was later proved incorrect in the monkey by Storm, working in de Waart's laboratory at Batavia (now Djakarta) in the 1930's.

It is true however that Einthoven complained to Lewis that it was sometimes difficult to distinguish between left ventricular hypertrophy and right (according to Lewis) bundlebranch block. This argument became the more stringent when it was found - several years after Einthoven's death, when Lewis' theory had already been refuted by Wilson's group in 1932 [121]-, that in a number of patients a temporary or permanent transition occurred from the pattern of left hypertrophy to the so-called right bundlebranch block. Much later again I noticed that, curiously enough in retrospect, Lewis himself in the 1925 edition of his book "Mechanism of the heart beat" (Ref. 89 p.137, figs. 89 and 90) had shown this transition of a "right bundlebranch block" into "left preponderance" with the complication of an (unrecognized) infarction in two ECG's of the same patient on successive days The similarity of the two patterns was noted but explained away; the clinical diagnosis was "aortic disease with febrile attack".

In conclusion, I want to stress again the growing friendship and trust between Einthoven and Lewis as shown in their letters and also the appreciation, even gratitude, of Einthoven for Lewis' work (fig.21). This was finally most clearly expressed in Einthoven's acceptance speech at the Nobel ceremony [59], see chapter 4).

On the other hand Lewis wrote in his letter of congratulation with the Nobel Prize: "You have given so much to Physiology and to medicine that the prize is but a small return; but I rejoice, and there will be many rejoicing with me that your great work has received this public recognition. No award could have given me greater satisfaction". To which Einthoven replied after his return from the U.S.A. (Jan. 3rd 1925): "Your words have touched me deeply. I owe so much to you --- You have given to Medicine at least as much as I have".

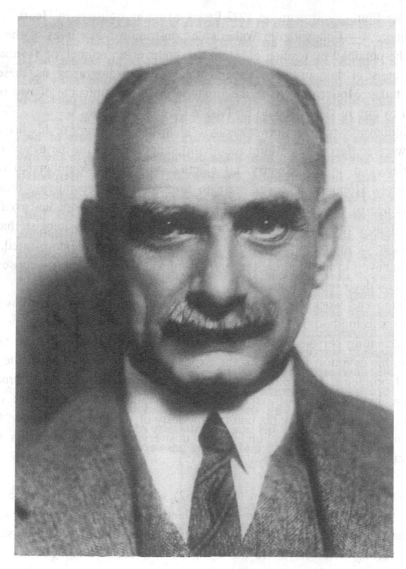

Figure 21.   *Sir Thomas Lewis in his forties with his penetrating look which I still remember. The portrait that Lady Lewis liked best as Dr. Hollman told me.*

After Einthoven's death in 1927 Lewis wrote an obituary in Heart [90], from which I quote: "--- Following up Waller's demonstration that curves of the heart beat can be obtained by leading off from the limbs of an animal, he [Einthoven] laid the basis of human and experimental electrocardiography as these are practised today. Modern electrocardiography is the direct outcome of two papers published by him in 1907 [should be 1906 [33] H.A.S.] and 1908 [38] ---".

"Einthoven's renown grew steadily and in the last years of his life many honours were conferred upon him; these culminated in 1924 in the award of the Nobel prize, and, in this country, his election to Foreign Membership of the Royal Society. Honours, however, were to him a smaller recompense than was the knowledge of the benefits which his long and arduous work had conferred upon his fellow men. To few scientists, perhaps to no physiologist, has the applied value of their discoveries been so abundantly been demonstrated, as it was to Einthoven in his lifetime, the strength of this demonstration surprised him and gave him deep satisfaction.

Einthoven's work will be remembered for all time for the greatness of his contributions to method. He himself will be remembered by those who knew him for his fascinating personality. A man of simple, almost humble habits, he was untiring in his devotion to work, to the exposition of his views and to the study of related problems. He awakened in both friends and associates a profound admiration, by his genius, by the charming simplicity and directness of his character, by his patience, by his unusual modesty of thought and manner, by his natural and unfailing courtesy, and by his unswerving devotion to truth in the most exacting sense ---".

Section 4. Frank N. Wilson (1890-1952) was for many years professor of medicine with the special assignment of electrocardiographic research and its application at the quiet city of Ann Arbor. In his later years he lived outside the town in a reconstructed farm. He was a mild-mannered, soft spoken man; he did not draw attention to himself but in due course he became known as the spiritual successor of both Einthoven and Lewis with a growing influence throughout the cardiological world. Especially so in Mexico and South America where he was one of the first promoters of scientific cooperation with the U.S.A.

As far as his relation to Einthoven and Lewis is concerned, he knew Lewis best, having been sent to him in wartime by the U.S. Army to study the soldier's heart syndrome. At that time he built close relations with Lewis, sharing his interest in electrocardiography and also in leisure activities such as observation (and photography) of birds. Scientifically Wilson may be viewed as a sort of middle man between Einthoven and Lewis, having in common with the former a preference for a physical and mathematical approach of electrocardiographic problems and with Lewis a clinical training and an interest in applying the outcome of experimental research in the clinical situation.

There were of course also differences between Wilson and both other men; as far as Einthoven is concerned, it is interesting to see various indications of the distinction between a "natural" physicist like Einthoven and a strictly disciplined physico-mathematical attitude acquired with great effort, like Wilson's. The latter attitude is the more striking, because it was and is alien to most clinicians. In any case, Wilson had a wide spread influence on electrocardiography, in the first place because of his theoretical views, but also, in retrospect even more so, by bringing to light the dilemma which in fact dated from Einthoven's work on the electrocardiographic signs of unilateral hypertrophy.

The dilemma namely, that while in normal electrocardiography Einthoven's simplified scheme of the equilateral triangle which represented the heart as a point (or rather dipole) in the centre continued to be of theoretical and practical importance, the examination of diseased hearts required attention to regional differences within the heart and therefore another way of exploration completing that by the standard leads. This was effectuated by Wilson and his group in the precordial "unipolar" leads which were considered "semi-direct leads" that is, almost equivalent to those from the cardiac surface. Wilson's six precordial electrodes were connected to a "central terminal" which itself was linked via resistors to all three limb electrodes and was considered (in fact, almost was) neutral, i.e. very little influenced by the heart beat. This was in 1932, five years after Einthoven's death. In 1942 the central terminal was modified by Goldberger for practical reasons. It soon became apparent that the most important and frequent use of the precordial leads lies in the field of coronary heart disease and Wilson devoted much time to the clinical and experimental study of this topic.

A bibliography with reprints of selected papers by Wilson and his group together with a concise biography can be found in the posthumous publication "Selected papers of Frank Wilson (1954)" [76]. The great majority of the selected papers had been previously published in wellknown cardiological journals; in the list of references these papers as far as they were quoted in the present volume are mentioned under the number of the original publication. Three aspects of this volume are of special interest in relation to Einthoven:

1)   one of the two previously unpublished papers by Wilson in this posthumous collection, is a belated supplementary and critical answer to Einthoven's letter of November 1921 [h], which at the time was thanked for by Wilson in cautious and non-committal terms. His later added critical comments, published after Wilson also had died, expressing the view, that "Einthoven's concept of myocardial contraction and the resulting electrocardiogram was true in the light of the then available evidence but incomplete in that it does not take full account of the difference (anatomical and physiological) between heart muscle and skeletal muscle nor of the fact that the skeletal muscle usually was examined in an dielectric medium (air) while the body surrounding the heart is a volume conductor".

2)   While several of Wilson's papers have some relation with concepts of Einthoven, in particular his scheme of the equilateral triangle, a few papers were written by Wilson with the explicit purpose to make Einthoven's ideas more accessible by giving additional information and spelling out what Einthoven had felt unnecessary to mention or explain.

3)   The inclusion of a few papers of a general and historical character - one of them intended for a partly non-medical audience [122] - are interesting and useful for understanding the development of electrocardiography (and ipso facto Einthoven's work and Wilson's addition to it). They supply also the clinical aspects and implications, which Einthoven usually avoided in his papers; this applies also to his final review of electrocardiography [61] posthumously published, and mentioned in chapter 4. Moreover the papers of a general nature by Wilson if taken together, replace to some extent the textbook which Wilson never wrote. I quote one of these papers (published in the American Heart Journal of 1930 [120], because it shows clearly Wilson's relation to Einthoven. It deals with the paper by Einthoven, Fahr and de Waart on the equilateral triangle [46].

About the construction of the manifest value of the heart vector from the standard leads: "This method is now well known --- nevertheless the principles do not appear to be generally appreciated. Having myself undertaken at one time a number of erroneous ideas regarding it --- it seems worthwhile to give a brief account of my difficulties in order that they may be avoided by others ---".

---

[h]   Einthoven's letter was in fact a reply to questions from Wilson relating to the equilateral triangle and the construction of the electrical axis from the corresponding deflections in the standard leads (text reprinted in: Selected papers on electrocardiography of Willem Einthoven, 1977 [101])

"Einthoven's original description of the method is a masterly one. All of the assumptions upon which it is based are clearly stated; the method is applied in the solution of several problems and its use is fully illustrated. It must be remembered however, that Einthoven was thoroughly familiar with electrical theory and mathematical physics --- Most electrocardiographers are neither mathematicians nor physicists."

From the limited correspondence between Einthoven and Wilson an important part is devoted to the double string galvanometer (two strings in optical series) which was constructed in Holland under Einthoven's supervision (see also pp. 36 and 117). It was intended for simultaneous recording of two leads or one lead with a phonocardiogram (fig.22).

I want to conclude this section by quoting Mrs Lepeschkin, Wilson's daughter, who was asked to talk about her father as well as Einthoven and Lewis. The latter two visited her home when she was still under 10 years of age. She read her paper [123] at a meeting on "Body surface mapping of cardiac fields" at Vermont (1972). She entitled her talk: "Three cardiologists from a mural" (together with Waller and others the three were painted on a wall in Mexico's Instituto de Cardiologia by Diego de Rivera).

Einthoven was described by Mrs Lepeschkin as "a well-built splendid, kindly-looking man with white hair, beard and moustache, soft-spoken, and I remember him saying very little socially ---. When he was in Ann Arbor it was rumoured that he had won the Nobel prize for his work - about 20 years after [doing this work]. However, he did not give credence to this and asked that no one accept it as truth, since in Holland a man had been giving parties and notices for a Nobel Prize which did not materialize". About Lewis: "I remember that I could not understand anything Sir Lewis said. He spoke behind his moustache in a kind of British clipped accent --- ." And about her father: "we often hear about the absent-minded professor, and my father was no exception. As a young child, I recall having to be quiet at meals because my father was reading at the table. Later in life he became a raconteur; but in his youth he was generally abstracted from realistic surroundings, because he was concentrating on what was important to him --- My father believed that leisure was important to the seeking of truth and that significant (in contrast to superficial) discoveries had taken place when individuals had conditions that gave them time for concentration and reflection ---."

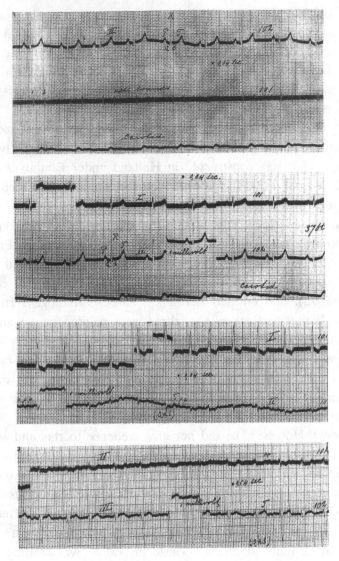

Figure 22. *Parts of a set of electrocardiograms made with 2 string galvanometers (numbers 101 and 102) which were coupled in order to take 2 leads simultaneously or one lead with phonocardiogram (with addition of optical record of carotid pulse). A) Normal person, Top to bottom: E.C.G., Lead II phonocardiogram, carotid pulse. B) Same normal, Lead I, Lead II, carotid pulse. C) Patient with left preponderance and atrial fibrillation: Leads I and II. D) Same patient: Lead II and III.*

Section 5. <u>Alexander Samojloff</u> (1867-1930) was a physiologist (pupil of Pavlov) who became an early pioneer of electrocardiography. His interest developed in his youth when he was fascinated by Lippmann's capillary electrometer and its records of the action of the exposed tortoise heart by Marey, and soon thereafter by Waller, who showed in addition that it was possible to register the heart's electrical activity in the intact animal and in man. Samojloff recalled this in 1929 when at the invitation of Paul White he read a paper about Einthoven at a meeting in the General Hospital of Massachussets at Boston [98]. He then told also about his own efforts to record the cardiac action curves with a capillary electrometer. However: "One day I obtained a copy of Einthoven's article in Pflüger's Archiv with records of the human heart. I understood that my technique was only a feeble attempt at the solution of a problem which in the hands of Einthoven was brought to the state of complete perfection. I spent hours examining these curves and asking myself: Who is this man and how does he obtain such results? Such sharpness distinguishing the curves of Einthoven was never obtained before. But such curves soon ceased to satisfy Einthoven --- He developed a method of correcting the curves and then I admired not only his technique but also his theoretical knowledge. These two accomplishments showed the essential features of Einthoven's talent. His mind worked like an instrument of precision --- Later we all could see that the subjects he chose for his investigations always lent themselves beautifully to precise measurements."

In 1904 Samojloff was at Paris during the summer vacation and wrote to Einthoven asking permission to come and see his laboratory; this visit took place a few weeks before the international physiological congress at Brussels. This event was the beginning of a correspondence (in German but quotations are presented here in English) and a friendship, which continued until Einthoven's death 23 years later. There was a rather long interruption due to World War I and the Russian revolution, but in 1921 the correspondence could be renewed and became busier than ever before, although for several years it had to be carried out through the intermediary of a friend in Dorpat (Estland), a former colleague of Samojloff at Kasan.

Samojloff himself was professor of physiology in Kasan and retained this position during the whole of his career in spite of all upheavals around him. Occasionally Samojloff wrote to Einthoven, that he had delivered a lecture or attended a meeting at Moscow, where his brother (who died before him) was professor of mineralogy. According to Krikler, who recently wrote several short papers about Samojloff [80,81,82,83], he was given the Lenin Prize. From Shostakovich' memoirs (as recorded by Volkov) we know however that this was not a safe protection against future disgrace.

Samojloff was the first to write a book or rather booklet on electrocardiography [96]; it was followed by many papers on the subject. However, although he was able to obtain excellent tracings for which he received compliments from Einthoven, and also displayed a good understanding of the development of electrocardiography, Samojloff's own contribution to the latter in his numerous papers was limited in scope as he was aware himself. In his correspondence with Einthoven electrocardiography and related subjects play a minor rôle, as compared to Einthoven's correspondence with Lewis. The letters from Samojloff express a need of friendship and of support (particularly in the postwar years) together with a feeling of intimacy based on common ideas and traits of character. From the latter Samojloff pointed out their mutual tendency to joking (very closely associated with basic seriousness). As an example of this love of joking (aptly called by Wiggers a naïve type of humour), Samojloff tells in his Boston memorial lecture on Einthoven mentioned above, that he wrote to Einthoven in 1923 recalling the first publication of electrocardiograms made with the string galvanometer 20 years earlier. He enclosed his congratulations to the galvanometer, which he asked Einthoven to read aloud to it, "since it can write, but can't read ". To which Einthoven replied: "I have carried out precisely your request and read to the galvanometer your letter. Apparently he listened and took in with pleasure and joy, all that you wrote --- but at the place where you said that he does not know how to read --- he cried: What, I can't read? It's a terrible lie. Do I not read all the secrets of the heart? I calmed him and advised him --- to work and to toil as much as he could for the benefit of humanity and not to think of gratitude ." [i] Something similar happened when Samojloff in October 1923 transmitted the greetings to the string galvanometer from his own large Edelmann galvanometer, adding that his small Edelmann model was "too ashamed to join because it was good for nothing". In passing it can be noted , that no indication can be found in the correspondence of Samojloff that suggests his possession of a string galvanometer either made at Leiden or in England. However it is true, that the University of Kasan is listed as an early customer of Cambridge Scientific Instruments (see also Burnett [9]). Perhaps the instrument

---

[i]   Quotation taken from Samojloff's paper. Einthoven did not make a copy of his answer, but only noted in Dutch: "Answered with a very friendly and for me, witty letter".

was bought on behalf of Prof. Mislawsky, a colleague of Samojloff at Kasan, who also was interested in the string galvanometer and had met Einthoven. He sometimes received Einthoven's greetings via Samojloff but there is no record of direct correspondence with Einthoven.

Another question that is not entirely clear, concerns the only known scientific difference of opinion between Samojloff and Einthoven. It is related with the Gaskell effect, mentioned earlier (chapter 4). This experiment was interpreted as a direct vagal effect upon the heart, whereas Einthoven demonstrated that in the Gaskell arrangement vagal stimulation resulted in contraction of the lungs and thereby stretching of the atrium, which in turn could be responsible for the unexpected change in demarcation current, which was observed. Krikler (The search for Samojloff [81]) reports that after the delayed publication of additional research by Samojloff in 1923 [97] Einthoven "conceded the honours". This is not quite correct; Einthoven wrote on October 2nd 1923 [in German]: "Although you did not convince me with your study of the positive change [of demarcation current] I have read it with much interest. I believe that you did not take sufficient account of the fact, that small changes in position may result in important variation of demarcation current. On the other hand it is true that Lepeschkin (whom Krikler quotes and who wrote 50 years after Einthoven's death) stated that subsequent work, in particular that with intracellular microelectrodes made clear that Einthoven's belief that there is a very close relation between electrical and mechanical response of muscle led to misinterpretation of tracings such as dealt with in Einthoven's correspondence with Wilson and the latter's posthumously published addition to it (see section 4 of this chapter). However, in my opinion this does not affect Einthoven's main point as put forward in his Harvey Lecture of 1924 [57] of "the complete parallelism" between electrical and mechanical activity of the myocardium, which ensures that "the medical practitioner stands on firm ground when building on the electrocardiogram" [as we have done ever since]. The - in retrospect less important - question of strict coincidence in time (especially onset) of the electrical and contractile activity is also discussed in the last section of this chapter.

In the years before the war, travelling was easy for Samojloff and he often made a journey through Italy, France or England in connection with an international congress of physiology. After the Russian revolution life became much more difficult. Nevertheless Samojloff chose to stay in Kasan, while his twin sons used an opportunity to leave the country. They went to the United States and with the help of their mother's brother who had settled near New York and some physiological friends of Samojloff himself, the boys managed to study in Boston and subsequently to build their career in the U.S.A. In this situation Samojloff renewed the correspondence with Einthoven who after hearing about the difficult situation in Kasan, offered a vacant assistant's position with the possibility of an additional income. Samojloff did not accept this offer but appealed the following year to Einthoven for help in arranging a trip to Holland which could be made possible by officially organising a lecture by Samojloff at Leiden.

It soon became apparent that the main wish of Samojloff was to travel from Holland to America and see his two sons; this required additional permits and arrangements partly through Samojloff's brother-in-law at New York but mostly with the help of Einthoven, who sent many letters to Dutch authorities in Berlin and inside Holland. While Samojloff was in America Einthoven even tried to enlist the help of a Dutch colleague staying in the U.S.A., to find a position there for Samojloff who for his part contacted his friends in Boston. Ultimately Samojloff decided to return to Kasan and to his wife with their two daughters. The following year Mrs Samojloff also managed to receive permission to visit America after a long struggle with the authorities; she stayed there for a year. The last part of the correspondence deals with the opportunity offered to Samojloff of visiting a neurophysiological laboratory in 1926; he decided to go to Magnus at Utrecht after the physiological congress in Stockholm. This again required a new permit, which Einthoven helped to obtain. On this occasion (end of 1926) Samojloff saw Einthoven at least once; at the end of this visit Einthoven gave Samojloff his signed portrait and intimated - as Samojloff reported in his Boston lecture already quoted - that this was probably their last encounter (which indeed it proved to be).

I conclude this section by quoting Samojloff once more about Einthoven: "First of all he is the creator of electrocardio-graphy; all methods proposed by him, his standardization, his electrodes, his three leads, his triangle, his terminology, all these are based on theory and at the same time are highly practical; they will all remain in electrophysiology, if not forever, at least for a long time".
--- "Later Einthoven demonstrated how to experiment with the currents of nerve fibres. He was the first to demonstrate the action current produced by heart contractions in the depressor nerve in its centripetal nerve fibres. He was the first to demonstrate the action current in the sympathetic nerve ---. He was given the greatest scientific honours and signs of distinction, including the Nobel Prize. But he remained the same simple, frank, direct man".

Section 6. A.V. Hill (1886-1977) started to study mathematics at Cambridge but became a physiologist at the suggestion of his teacher Sir Walter Fletcher. His main research concerned muscular contraction and especially its production of heat for which he received the Nobel Prize in 1922, jointly with biochemist Meyerhof. Later he was able to measure the heat production by nerve action. He was professor of Physiology at Manchester and London successively and member of the Royal Society since 1918. A very interesting review of his work on the heat production of muscle and nerve together with a bibliography, 1909-1964, was provided by Hill himself in Annual Review of Physiology 1965, entitled "Trails and trials in physiology" [71]. In many ways his career and scientific approach resembled those of Einthoven, although their start was different. From the correspondence it is evident that there was also a similarity of character and life style (e.g. simplicity, frankness and frugality). Their correspondence differed from the others in that it started late (in 1922) but soon led to friendship and intimacy. It was also unusual that it was initiated by Einthoven: the latter wanted to repeat Hill's experiments on muscular heat production.

Einthoven had already ordered in December 1920 from the instrument maker Wilson who supplied A.V. Hill, "a thermopile with many couples and mounted in a suitable chamber as described by you [Hill]". In spite of a reminding letter from Einthoven there was no answer. Einthoven therefore appealed to Hill for advice. The answer from Hill came on Feb. 14, 1922: "--- I am sorry you have been unable to get a thermopile from Mr Wilson, I cannot understand his delay ---, but I know that he has been very busy and possibly he has forgotten all about it. I am not sure however, that the instruments which he makes are really as good as the ones which we make here much more laboriously --- and as I have an instrument here which I do not really require, at least at present, I am sending it to you in a separate parcel and hope you will accept it and find useful in your experiments". [Follow instructions how to use it]. There is no further record or published article by Einthoven on this matter.

Subsequently reprints of papers were exchanged - from Leiden the bound collections of reprints ("Onderzoekingen physiologisch laboratorium Leiden") - and on Sept. 18, 1923 Hill sent a letter of thanks after having visited Einthoven's laboratory. In the same letter Hill asked Einthoven if he had any objections if Gasser from the U.S.A. who worked with Hill at that moment, would take up the subject of the relation between mechanical and electrical action in skeletal muscle. A subject, which Einthoven and Hill had discussed; Einthoven had announced it as one of his planned investigations. In the heart muscle this topic had been examined repeatedly by Einthoven and his co-workers; now this ought to be performed in skeletal muscle. It should be noted that Gasser was already a well known physiologist at that time who received the Nobel prize 20 years later together with Erlanger. Einthoven answered graciously that he had no objections (no copy, but a few lines scribbled on Hill's letter).

After a letter from Hill who had moved to London requesting new reprints of Einthoven's papers because he had given those received earlier to the library at Manchester (Jan. 9, 1924), follows a letter of thanks for the reprints, which had been sent accordingly.

We find in Einthoven's archive also a hand-written text of Einthoven's introduction of Hill as speaker at an unspecified meeting at Leiden in April 1924 when he stayed for a few days at Einthoven's home. In July and August 1924 a correspondence follows on how to sail to America: on what ship and in which class, but in any case intending to do it together. In fact they went on the same boat to New York but Einthoven returned some weeks later than Hill. Mrs Einthoven and her sister accompanied Einthoven on his journey but they made an independent tour together in that country.

By now their friendship was cemented and Hill's letter of Aug. 4, 1924 begins with: "Dear Einthoven, I pay you the English compliment of addressing you without a prefix". [j] The tone of the letter though sometimes dealing with very practical matters such as prices and dates of ships, became more intimate. Even almost lyrical, when Hill on April 7, 1925 thanked Mrs Einthoven for her "extra-ordinary hospitality during the meeting of the British Physiological Society at Leiden" --- Every single one of the visitors was filled with enthusiasm for the perfect hospitality provided --- The magnificence of your reception of us was equalled only by the sincerity and simplicity and informality and goodwill which we found everywhere. Please believe how very, very grateful we all are --- and shall remain. (N.B. The repetitive "and" was replaced by + every time; the occasion was the first meeting of the Physiological Society on foreign soil, which took place at Leiden on Einthoven's invitation after he had been elected a honorary member of that society).

There were several letters with communications of a scientific character such as the announcement by Hill that he had measured the heat production of nerve (May 1, 1926). Soon afterwards Hill sent a description of Brownian movements in his extremely sensitive records and a letter on Sept. 2, 1926 asking

---

[j]   All preceding letters were headed: Dear Professor Einthoven.

if Einthoven agreed to Hill's conclusion from them. This was answered in the affirmative by Einthoven on Sept. 7th, giving the pertinent references. Shortly afterwards Einthoven sent an antiquarian copy of the exhausted thesis on Brownian movements by Mrs de Haas-Lorentz in its German translation of 1912.

Most of the important topics in the correspondence are reflected in Hill's obituary of Einthoven in Nature [70]. I quote a few lines, which bear testimony to Hill's keen observation and his sincere admiration of Einthoven: "Einthoven's investigations cover a wide range, but they are all notable for the same characteristic - the mastery of physical technique which they show. Einthoven, in spite of his medical training and his office, was essentially a physicist, and the extraordinary value of his contributions to physiology, and therewith indirectly to medicine, emphasizes the way in which an aptitude - in Einthoven's case a genius - for physical methods can aid in the solution of physiological problems ---". And on the string galvanometer: "In 1909 he published the first complete description of the instrument, while in the last few years, employing fibres of almost ultramicroscopic size working in a high vacuum, he has succeeded together with his son, an electrical engineer, in recording potential changes of frequencies in the order of 100.000 per second. It may be mentioned also that recently, by means of fibres of extreme thinness he was able to register directly, and with very little distortion, sound waves of more than 10.000 vibrations per second ---. Of the more personal side of Einthoven's life one might write of the grace, beauty, and simplicity of his character --- It was a wonderful thing to be his guest and to enjoy the delightful hospitality of his home". Such an occasion arrived in 1923 after a congress at Tübingen: "We arranged to meet at a station in northern Germany and to travel the last part of the journey together --- He came literally running along the platform to meet me, seized my bag out of my hand and carried it to the carriage, where he had kept me the best seat and made me feel that whatever the difference of our age and position, I was from that moment his honoured guest". (N.B. Hill was younger by 26 years but won a Nobel Prize two years before Einthoven).

Section 7. C.J. Wiggers (1883-1963). Wiggers' father was a German immigrant, who left the parental farm in Holstein (northern Germany) because of economic circumstances. Carl Wiggers was born in America and found his wife there, whose father also was an immigrant from Holstein. For 35 years Wiggers was professor of physiology at Western Reserve University Medical School, Cleveland. Shortly after his retirement he became editor of the new journal for basic research in cardiology, which split off from Circulation as Circulation Research. Probably he will be best remembered because of his experimental research on the dynamics of heart and circulation in connection with clinical problems such as those in valvular heart disease.

Wiggers met Einthoven for the first time at the physiological congress of Edinburgh (1923), and subsequently during Einthoven's lecture tour in America, where the latter also visited Cleveland and stayed at Wiggers' home. They met again in 1926 when Wiggers went to see some European laboratories in Belgium, Germany and Holland, before going to the physiological congress at Stockholm. This occasion marked also the beginning of their limited correspondence: on Feb. 23, 1926 Wiggers wrote a letter to Einthoven asking if he could come and visit him in his laboratory before the Stockholm congress. This was arranged by Einthoven who also invited Wiggers to his home. Wiggers was deeply impressed by Einthoven's personality and his approach to scientific problems. He made a study of Einthoven's writings and his rôle in the development of electrocardiography [k], which enabled him to write an excellent paper at the centenary of Einthoven's birth in Circulation Research [119]. A few years earlier Wiggers had already given some details of Einthoven's visit to Cleveland and his own impressions when visiting Leiden, in his autobiography "Reminiscences and Adventures in Circulation Research." [118] In this book it is described, that during Einthoven's visit to Cleveland Wiggers showed him records of intraventricular and aortic pressure registered simultaneously with the electrocardiogram, that did not seem to agree with Einthoven's evidence of the strict coincidence of mechanical and electrical signs of myocardial activity. "Einthoven frankly admitted the apparent differing evidence and pointed out that investigators should perhaps spend more energy in attempts to harmonize differences than to gather more and more experimental evidence in favour of a previous conclusion. He said: The Truth is all that matters; what you or I may th6ink is inconsequential." In the same book Wiggers' visit to Leiden also is described. I quote some observations relating to the home of the Einthoven's and the physiological laboratory: "Their home life was simple but edified by the professor's genial personality and the wife's motherly solicitude" --- "Einthoven's research laboratory was small and unique. In

---

[k]   Wiggers also mentioned having studied de Waart's biography of Einthoven where Wiggers doubtless obtained part of his information. In retrospect one wonders, if strict coincidence of electrical and mechanical events can occur at all, seeing that single cell potentials have been measured for the last 40 years while mechanical effects still require the cooperation of many cells, to be detectable.

a large room covered by a glass canopy one saw five cement pillars arising from great depth in the soil. To these the galvanometers could be transported by means of derricks attached to rollers on heavy beams".

"Einthoven deserves the gratitude of every patient in whom a diagnosis of a cardiac disorder has been aided through electrocardiography. His right to fame is not dimmed by occasional attempts of his disgruntled colleagues (Wiggers was perhaps thinking of Kraus and Nicolai, see chapter 7) to minimize his accomplishments as a physicist, a physiologist and a discerning cardiologist".

From Wiggers' paper on Einthoven, written 100 years after the latter's birth, I do not need to quote very much, having already quoted Wiggers' account of the mutual visits. I want to mention however, that Wiggers was one of the very few writers on Einthoven's work, who paid particular attention to the early stage of the development of electrocardiography around 1895 before the string galvanometer was constructed (but the term electrocardiogram had already been coined). Wiggers wrote: "In 1889 A.D. Waller had reported that electrical currents generated during the heart beat could be tapped from the body surface and recorded by capillary electrometer. Human electrocardiography may thus be said to have been born in Oxford (should be London!), England. However, since Waller went to great pains to rule out any possible clinical application of the procedure, this proved to be a stillbirth. Waller's conclusion need not surprise us if we view again the wholly unsatisfactory character of his records --- it is at this point that we gain a good insight into Einthoven's genius - a human trait that Carlyle has defined as "the ability to take infinite pains". Einthoven, like several other physiologists, was naturally impelled to repeat Waller's significant observations. Instead of merely using such capillary electrometers as were available in his laboratory, he first tested their physical characteristics and found that their performance could be materially improved by attention to minor expedients, including the resistance of the external circuits. --- As shown by the sharp pike alone, these records were immeasurably superior to those recorded by Waller.

Meanwhile, Einthoven and Burch had independently devised procedures by which capillary electrometer records could be corrected. --- Thus, the true characteristics of the human cardiac action potentials were established by Einthoven even before the beginning of the present century ---".

After mentioning Einthoven's theoretical studies culminating in his famous paper with Fahr and de Waart about the equilateral triangle [46], Wiggers added a series of remarks about Einthoven's personality. At the time of Wiggers' first contact with Einthoven (at the physiological congress at Edinburgh of 1923),

"Einthoven had already reached the zenith of his career as attested by the bestowal of an honorary doctorate degree by the University of Edinburgh. Nevertheless new acquaintances recognized only a modest, cordial, and earnest man --- I was particularly impressed by his greeting of younger persons --- I later learned that he was equally generous in showing "unimportant people" through the laboratory and, if requested, offered them advice in matters pertaining to electrocardiography."

It is tempting to quote much more of this shrewd and at times moving account but I think the summing up of Einthoven's character by Wiggers will suffice: "In various memorials, Einthoven's friends and colleagues praised his modesty, his gracious manners, his unpretentious habits, his natural curiosity, his warm hospitality, his zeal for work, his resilient mind and his devotion to the search for truth. He exemplifies to us all, the need of remaining humble in the face of the vast ocean of ignorance that still confronts us. "

Apart from the letters concerning Wiggers' visit to Leiden there are in Einthoven's archive only two others to mention: on June 28, 1927 Wiggers asked permission to use Einthoven's picture as a frontispiece to a book on electrocardiography he had promised to write and to dedicate the book to Einthoven; he also asked for a picture of the newest type of galvanometer which Wiggers had seen at Leiden in order to use it as illustration. The following answer came from Einthoven on September 5th, 1927: "My dear Dr Wiggers, I have been operated on, and am lying in bed since several months. This is the cause, that you did not receive earlier an answer on your kind letter of June 28th. Now I am trying to dictate the letter from my bed. The three favours you ask for are for me three great honours. So I agree with much pleasure indeed. You will find enclosed two photo's of the new models of the galvanometer both of them devised by my son: engineer W.F. Einthoven. The smaller one represents two samples of the galvanometer, arranged in optical series and so firmly and solidly fixed to one another, that they constitute one single mechanical piece. The coupling of the two galvanometers to one mechanical entity has been a suggestion of Frank N. Wilson at Ann Arbor. A limited number of the new type galvanometers has been commercially available at "Instrumenthandel Salm, Keizersgracht 642-644, Amsterdam, Holland."
With kind regards
Yours sincerely,
W. Einthoven.

Einthoven died a few weeks later, on September 29th, 1927. Probably this letter was sent unsigned and without corrections. On the copy an unidentified hand had registered the photographs that were included.

Chapter 7.

Additional evaluations of Einthoven's work (by not personally acquainted authors) including Johansson (chairman Nobel Prize Committee) together with comments on Kraus and Nicolai; furthermore Burch and De Pasquale; Katz and Hellerstein; Shapiro; Cooper (Sections 1 and 4-7).

Some correspondence and arrangements concerning production of the string galvanometer in particular with Edelmann and Ebert together with a comparison of Einthoven's work to that of Ader (Sections 2 and 3).

In this chapter some additional evaluations of Einthoven's work are reviewed in the light of the data presented in precedent chapters. It will be seen, that these appraisals provide information about Einthoven's work, which has to be examined critically, as there is a wide divergency in factual accuracy and in carefulness of quotations. In contrast to chapters 5 and 6 none of the authors mentioned here could draw on previous personal acquaintance with Einthoven. For sake of clarity, this chapter is divided into 7 sections.

Section 1. The first paper to be discussed is the statement on Einthoven's work by Professor J.E. Johansson, chairman of the committee for the Nobel prize of physiology and medicine in 1924. As could be expected, his evaluation is based on a very thorough study of Einthoven's writings and those of his contemporaries working in the same field. Only now and then it becomes clear that Johansson was a pure physiologist, not "essentially a physicist" (A.V. Hill) like Einthoven himself. The publication by the Nobel Foundation in 1965 [75] contains also a short biography of Einthoven which brings no new information. The contemporary writings offering other descriptions and explanations of the electrocardiogram [in the case of Waller as well as Kraus and Nicolai showing their preference to maintain their own terminology and choice of leads] may perhaps seem to be dismissed too lightly by Johansson in the following words: "It is unnecessary --- to consider the interpretations proposed by other investigators, as Einthoven's concept is the only one which is tenable". Nevertheless Johansson's paper appears to be soundly based on the published facts and his conclusion seems justified. More information about Waller was given in chapter 6, section 2. About Kraus and Nicolai can be told that they not only failed to recognize the importance of the three standard leads, but thought that one lead only should suffice. (Kraus, Nicolai, Meyer in 1914 [79]: "Jedenfalls halten wir es unten den gegebenen Verhältnissen unbedingt für wissenschaftlich exacter, eine Ableitung erschöpfend durch zu arbeiten, als wahllos mit allen möglichen Ableitungen sein Glück zu versuchen." ("In our opinion it is scientifically more correct to investigate one single lead exhaustively than to try out all possible leads at random"). This quotation from a paper appearing in the same journal (Pflüger's Archiv) as Einthoven's publication on the equilateral triangle and electrical axis one year earlier [46], shows the incompetence of the authors who attack Einthoven pretending that some of his conclusions were incorrect. It is likely, that Wiggers (see end of chapter 6) thought of Kraus and Nicolai when writing of "occasional attempts of disgruntled colleagues to minimize his [Einthoven's] accomplishments".[a]

Johansson characterized Einthoven's work as a threefold invention.

First: discovery of the true electrocardiogram by correcting the capillary electrometer tracing and subsequently - in order to make the examination widely applicable - the construction of the string galvanometer which directly registers the true tracing without correction.

Second: ascertaining the different characteristics of the electrocardiogram, i.e. the individual variations within the framework of a general, broadly similar pattern and on the other hand the pathological changes which do not identify an individual person, but a disease or a change caused thereby such as hypertrophy. In this category is also placed the identification of the P wave as expression of atrial and the QRST complex indicating ventricular activity.

Third: the discovery of the mechanism of the electrocardiogram. The latter is based on the one side on the different shapes of the three leads in one person and their relation to the total electrical activity of the heart as shown in the scheme of the equilateral triangle. On the other side on the anatomy of the conduction system which allows impulses to reach the left and right ventricular myocardium at about the same time. Johansson emphasizes that in 1908 Einthoven was the first to use the knowledge about the conduction system in his concept, whereas Lewis was responsible for determining the high conduction

---

[a]   It should be added that Nicolai showed a much more sympathetic side of his militancy in his fight for pacifism and individual freedom, which forced him to leave Germany for South America. There he ultimately abandoned cardiology for sociology (Krikler [80])

velocity in the specific system as compared with the myocardium and the consequences thereof for the spread of excitation.

In most respects however, Johansson saw Lewis' work essentially as a confirmation of Einthoven's concept, although he recognized that the work of Lewis had been important for its general acceptance. On the latter point he appears to concur with Einthoven himself whose reference to Lewis during his speech at the Nobel Prize Ceremony was mentioned in chapters 4 and 6. Whether Johansson had been inclined to follow the suggestion of Hill (see my edition of the Einthoven-Lewis correspondence [102]) that the Nobel Prize should be awarded to Einthoven and Lewis together, will probably never be known. Neither, why the Nobel Committee as a whole, which certainly will have considered the possibility of a joint award, could not agree to do so. The Nobel Prize was awarded to Einthoven for the "discovery of the mechanism of the electrocardiogram". A formulation, which appears more diplomatic (avoiding all problems about Ader and Edelmann etc.) than adequate to express Einthoven's merits for electrocardiography, cardiology and cardiac patients.

Section 2. Correspondence and some additional information about commercial production of the string galvanometer, in particular correspondence with Edelmann and Ebert.

In contrast to the evaluation by Johansson, the assessment by firms engaged in making instruments understandably was based on commercial considerations. In every case the initiative to this kind of correspondence was taken by Einthoven, in some instances encouraged by physiologists such as Waller at London and Engelmann at Berlin (formerly at Utrecht). Most of the German and British firms however were not interested, at least not for the moment. Later the Dutch firms Kipp and subsequently Salm constructed special types of the string galvanometer (see below). Ultimately the string galvanometer was chiefly manufactured by Edelmann from Munich and by Cambridge Scientific Instruments later called Cambridge Instruments Company, from London; subsequently also by Hindle (New York) together with the Cambridge Instrument Company of America and finally also by Eiga in Holland (see later in this chapter).

The correspondence with Cambridge Scientific Instruments in the Einthoven archive was used by J. Burnett for his paper on "the origins of the electrocardiograph as a clinical instrument", which formed part of a symposium organized by the Wellcome Institute and was published in Medical History (1985 [9]).

More than 30 years earlier the history of the Cambridge string galvanometer had already been described by S.L. Barron ("The development of the electrocardiograph", 1952 [3]). Barron's booklet includes a biography of Willem Einthoven which in spite of a few incorrect details, gives the impression to be based on inside information; perhaps from the physicist Bergansius, who joined Einthoven's staff in 1911 and was Barron's chief interlocutor.

Special attention will be given here to the correspondence with Ebert and Edelmann Sr and Jr (father and son); the father being head of the firm, but also holding the title of Professor like his friend Ebert. The correspondence is written in German, but my quotations are given in English. In keeping with other parts of the correspondence (see Burnett [9]) the letters to Edelmann show that Einthoven was not primarily aiming at financial gains, but at recognition of his work (like he was always careful himself to give others their due credit) and above all, a satisfactory use of his galvanometer.

This correspondence begins with several letters about technical matters which I do not need to discuss here; but then follows a letter from Einthoven to Edelmann's friend Prof. Ebert (Jan. 30, 1907): "Thank you for sending me your reprint. You say on p. 553 that I have refined the string galvanometer devised by Ader. One can have different opinions on Ader's merits with relation to the string galvanometer and I don't want to fight about that now. As you know I mentioned Mr Ader in my first publication and at the same time I have described in a few words his instrument - a receiver to be used in telegraphy.

In connection with your assertion, that Dr M. Edelmann Jr likewise is responsible for a refinement of the string galvanometer I want to make a comment and ask a question".

The main argument of this comment is that Edelmann [b] wrote to Einthoven who had sent him a reprint of his 1903 publication on the string galvanometer accompanied by a letter with more details, that it was a pity that no patent could be taken out because the invention had been fully published. (The same remark was also made by Horace Darwin from Cambridge Scientific Instruments, see Burnett [9]). Subsequently Einthoven was asked to send his conditions and his suggestions for possible ameliorations. Einthoven did so; he proposed to construct also a smaller instrument with a permanent magnet, which would have no need of cooling by water. Its sensitivity would be 10 times less than his own instrument

---

[b] The letters from the Edelmann Institute were mostly signed by Edelmann Jr; the final letter by both of them.

with an electromagnet, but that could suffice if the construction was good. The answer from Edelmann Jr was, that the construction of a simpler instrument was being undertaken.

However, less than a year later, on Febr. 17, 1905 Edelmann had taken out legal protection (Musterschütz) in his own name for a small model of the string galvanometer. In 1906 he published this construction as his own design. Einthoven's question now was the following: If he would publish this state of affairs in the context of a subsequent paper on the string galvanometer, should he then mention the name of Ebert together with Edelmann or was Ebert going to change his opinion on the merits of Edelmann? In retrospect this letter appears to demonstrate that Einthoven had a naïve side not only in his kind of humour - as Wiggers remarked - but also in other respects. It is not surprising that Ebert in his answer (on paper of the Physical Institute of the Technical College at Munich) showed himself a faithful supporter of Edelmann Sr and Jr and agreed that his own name should be mentioned together with Edelmann and the Edelmann Institute.

A copy of this letter apparently was sent to the Edelmanns, who answered together with indignation, that nobody could object to having his name being connected with Edelmann. The proposals from Einthoven were said to be too vague or, alternatively, reverting to the old concept of Ader. Moreover, under German law the "Musterschütz" which Edelmann had obtained was said to be totally different from a patent. The former applied only to a distinct model (designed by Edelmann in this case), based on a known principle (presumably meaning Ader's).

To cut a long story short: Edelmann concluded, that they now felt justified to break the agreement with Einthoven, who could contact any other firm which only would have to respect Edelmann's legal protection rights. No further payments were going to be made. This is the end of the Edelmanns correspondence in the Einthoven's archive.

The arrangement with Cambridge Scientific Instruments which aimed at the distribution of string galvanometers in Great Britain and the United States was continued; only the payment of 10% to Einthoven for each instrument sold was lowered to 5%, because other firms would also construct string galvanometers. The U.S. market was mainly supplied by C.S.I. American's Hindle, who had ties with H.B. Williams at New York; the latter in turn was well acquainted with Einthoven and had designed an improved version of the Edelmann type of string galvanometer. In Holland a brief series of firms successively was occupied with the construction, in particular of special types such as the coupling of two galvanometers in optical series (see chapter 6). Before or shortly after the end of Einthoven's life a new firm "Eiga" (from Einthoven galvanometer) under the supervision of Einthoven's then chief mechanic de Groot constructed a somewhat simplified but otherwise authentic model which was used for example in the medical clinic at Leiden, where I worked with this instrument in the 1930's. For the sake of completeness I mention the French (Boulitte) model of string galvanometer, which was constructed at about the end of Einthoven's life and reached the European hospitals (including Leiden University Hospital) in the early 1930's.

The conclusion can be drawn that Einthoven could not cope with the arrangement of commercial or financial matters. More important: that his trust in other people's honesty and sincerity was shaken and that he felt hurt, because a commercial firm did not take his own honesty for granted. In retrospect one can also wonder if Edelmann (apart from wanting to keep his money) also felt hurt by Einthoven's lack of appreciation for his work. Edelmann certainly did not fully understand that the original string galvanometer had been constructed in the workshop of Einthoven's laboratory and under his own supervision; in fact he asked Einthoven repeatedly to make sure that the original constructor would not make any more instruments and sell them. It can be safely assumed that also at London the impression was that Einthoven disposed of a special constructing team besides his regular staff. (figs. 23 and 24).

Section 3. Einthoven and Ader.

It appears justified to conclude with de Waart and the physicists he consulted [109], that apart from the galvanometer of Ewing [65] using two strings which was published a few years before Ader (see below), the principle of a conducting wire in a magnetic field moving when a current passes through it, had been known from Faraday's time if not earlier, that is three quarters of a century before Ader. Equalizing all possible instruments which use that principle is perhaps just as meaningless as to put a primitive horse cart on a par with a Rolls Royce, because they both ride on wheels. [c]

---

[c]   Burnett is more detailed and also more polite in his paper mentioned above, by pointing out which elements of Ader's galvanometer (an inappropriate name, as Burnett proves by saying that it was not a measuring instrument) and Einthoven's string galvanometer had in common (such as light weight and swiftness of response). But: "Ader's galvanometer was very different from Einthoven's. In particular, it was less sensitive".

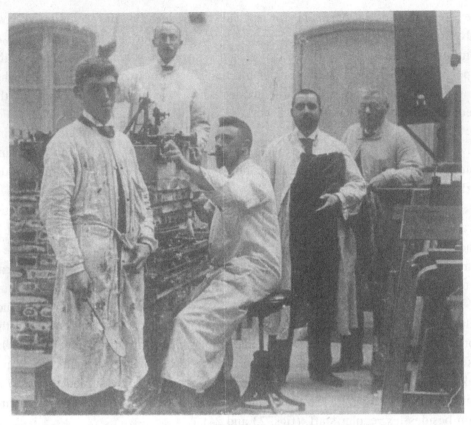

Figure 23   *Einthoven's technical staff, probably around 1900, at the time of construction of the first string galvanometer (no date recorded). Chief technician van der Woerd, who retired in 1906, in the rear at right.*

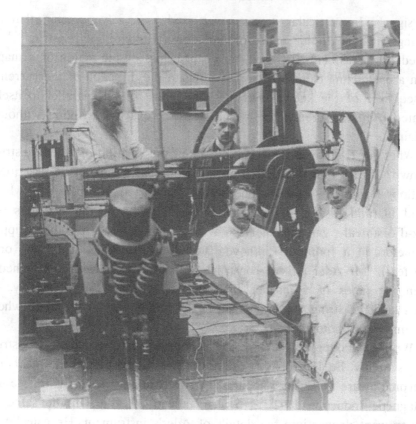

Figure 24. *Technical team of Einthoven (presumably a few years later than preceding photograph). Van der Woerd now at left, again at the rear. Note the changes in the technical staff.*

This comparison is not meant to belittle Ader's instrument. The latter answered its purpose beautifully and Ader himself, if he was Clément Ader (no initials were given in the original publication (1) nor in the subsequent papers by Rossel [95] but Cooper's reference list [10] calls him C. Ader) was a famous engineer. He became a millionaire through his inventions in the field of electricity; in France he was later known as "father of aviation" because of his attempts at flying, by which he is said to have lost his fortune.

In any case, neither Ader [1] nor Rossel [95] saw Ader's instrument in any other light than that of an extraordinary rapid receiver of submarine telegraphic

Morse signals. In particular it was never used as a galvanometer, that is for measuring currents. In his paper on "un nouvel appareil enregistreur" [1] Ader described his instrument as "based on the principle of the action of a magnetic field on a conducting element --- . According to the direction of the current and in consequence of the known laws the wire tends to shift parallel to itself ---" (translated from the French text which gives an exact description without any false claims).

What did Einthoven think himself about the relation of Ader's instrument to his own? In his first publication on the string galvanometer he described the calculations leading to this instrument (see chapter 3), by means of which he expected to (and in fact did) achieve a combination of the swiftness of the Duprez-d'Arsonval galvanometer and the sensitivity of the Lippmann electrometer. In a footnote Einthoven added (as translated from the original French text): "Mr Ader already constructed an instrument with a stretched wire between the poles of a magnet. This was a receiver for telegraphy. Using feather's quill the string was broadened in the middle, i.e. at the place where its movements were photographed [29,1].

Writing about the details of the string galvanometer's construction (Pflüger's Archiv. Bd 130, 1909 [40]) Einthoven mentioned that in the meantime he had become aware of Ewing's apparatus for recording tracings of magnetization (in: Magnetic Induction 1892 [65]), 5 years ahead of Ader. In the same paper Einthoven went deeper into the details of Ader's instrument. He calculated the latter's sensitivity, if used as a galvanometer, as 1:100.000 compared to the string galvanometer. Einthoven did not discuss Ader again, obviously feeling that his own instrument and Ader's were different enough in construction and intended use, to avoid any further association or confusion.

Why took some later authors the rôle of Ader as precursor of Einthoven seriously? From those who reserved a place for Ader in electrocardiographic history I discuss first the well known book on the History of electrocardiography by Burch and De Pasquale (1964 [7]) and second, Katz and Hellerstein in their chapter on electrocardiography of "Circulation of the blood; Men and Ideas" (eds. Fishman and Dickinson Richards, also from 1964 [77]).

Section 4. <u>Burch and De Pasquale</u> [7] write rather little about Ader and mention Einthoven's ignorance of Ader's instrument during his own construction of the string galvanometer. They also state: "Einthoven will always be remembered as the inventor of the string galvanometer and the father of electrocardiography".[d] Nevertheless and in spite of the difference in purpose and design, they talk of Ader's "string galvanometer" and put his instrument on the list of historic events important to electrocardiography. Perhaps this came about through the double authorship of their book or the relation of Burch with Cohn of the Rockefeller Institute who was the first to introduce a string galvanometer (made by Edelmann) into the U.S.A. This instrument was later acquired by Burch; a letter from Cohn concerning its use during 30 years was printed by Burch and De Pasquale. This letter does not mention Ader however, only the use of the Edelmann apparatus in New York and its improved counterpart designed by Prof. H.B. Williams and constructed by Hindle.

Besides wrongly representing Ader as a pioneer of electrocardiography, Burch and De Pasquale also assert that Einthoven was aided by the mathematician Kluyver (mis-spelled as Kluyner) because Einthoven was "weak in mathematics". Presumably this information is based on Barron's brief biography of Einthoven [3] where Kluyver is mentioned and Einthoven is said to be "not strong in mathematics". The latter perhaps refers to Einthoven's early period at Leiden around 1890 when he studied differential and integral calculus from Lorentz' book. The Einthoven correspondence contains only one small note from Kluyver and de Waart's monograph does not mention him. In conversation with the present author de Waart described Kluyver's help as unimportant.

Section 5. <u>Katz and Hellerstein</u> [77] take a further step by claiming that "Ader invented a new type of galvanometer now known as string galvanometer ---". They then introduce Willem Einthoven as "the founder of modern electrocardiography" but "his fundamental early achievement was the recognition of the potential of Ader's new, elegant galvanometer and his own construction of an improved and more sensitive modification of this machine". They quote the already mentioned paper "Un nouveau galvanomètre" (1901 [29]) and the subsequent paper (1903 [31]) in German on the recorded electrocardiograms. But it will be clear from the foregoing that Einthoven's announcement of the new galvanometer was a discussion of a construction based on calculation, <u>not</u> on imitation of Ader's instrument and/or improvement thereof.

---

[d] In a letter of Sept.18, 1984 to the present author Burch used more glowing terms for praising Einthoven (and Lewis): "There is no doubt that both were outstanding people, and that Einthoven, of course, will remembered forever. His electrocardiography will be with us, I think, for many centuries to come".

Is this an example of a quotation without careful reading of the original or a distrust of Einthoven's account? In any case, to speak of Ader's "elegant galvanometer" is a misnomer because Ader's instrument was neither a galvanometer nor particularly elegant, with its thickening of the string in the middle by quill in order to increase visibility.

There is more, because Katz and Hellerstein demand attention (justified of course) to Waller and the early pioneers of electrophysiology whom they discuss extensively; they feel that "the brilliant success of Einthoven's instrument, and the world renown which came to him on the basis of this achievement pushed into the background the basic discoveries of earlier physiologists upon which his own work actually rested". In their view this was particularly true of Augustus D. Waller, but Waller's own attitude proved "generous" by accepting Einthoven's frank acknowledgement, that "his own work was the direct continuation of mine, and that his string galvanometer was invented with the direct object of providing a more adequate recording of the human electrocardiogram than was afforded by the capillary electrometer". This is true indeed although by no means the complete truth. Katz and Hellerstein do not explain, why speaking the truth is called generous. It would have been interesting if they had defined what elements from Waller's work and that of the other physiologists still could be found in the current electrocardiography of 1964 (the year of their publication) as compared to Einthoven's research and methodology.

Einthoven's correction of the Lippmann tracings in the early 1890's is mentioned by Katz and Hellerstein but not recognized - like Johansson did - as the discovery of the true electrocardiogram. In fact, Katz and Hellerstein contend that in the early phase (the 1890's) of Einthoven's research, which "seems methodical and uninspiring compared to later events, emphasis was placed on the definition of component parts of the tracings and no link can be found with his publications of later thoughts on vector analysis, the effect of position etc". The meaning of this sentence is not quite clear, but the last part of it is certainly not correct (see below).

In his paper with de Lint of 1900 [28] Einthoven summarized his work of the 1890's with the Lippmann electrometer in a report on the electrocardiograms of 17 normals and 2 patients with aortic insufficiency. The influence of the position of the body and of accelerated heart rate (these were the first electrocardiograms taken after exercise) were discussed as well as the significance of the P.Q.R.S.T. deflections (at this moment it seemed possible that not only P but also Q belonged to the atrial complex). Moreover both the differences and the general similarity in shape of the ECG in various leads were studied. The first phonocardiographic paper ever was published in 1894 [23], including tracings of aortic insufficiency both experimental and clinical. One year earlier Einthoven already told the Dutch Medical Association about two new clinical methods with great promise for the future: electrocardiography and phonocardiography [21]. Meanwhile physical research on the Lippmann electrometer was published as well as some papers about quite different subjects (on bronchial constriction in asthma nervosum [19], on optical illusions [20] and on the physiology of the pharynx [27]). Is all this "uninspiring"? The term "methodical" can indeed be said to apply to this part as well as all other parts of Einthoven's work.

I want to discuss two more papers before making some concluding remarks. These papers were published fairly recently and do not claim to reveal the entire historical development of electrocardiography or electrophysiology. However, they cannot be said to be entirely free from pretension: they both try to show unknown aspects of Einthoven and his work and to take a fresh look on him; apparently he was considered a legendary figure, who probably would reveal himself differently on closer scrutiny.

Section 6. The first of the last papers to discuss is by E. Shapiro [100] and called "Willem Einthoven's fortuitous invention" (1977). It gives the facts as they are except a few minor errors, but it fails in their interpretation. The main argument is that Einthoven initially was interested in ophthalmology and optical illusions, planning to become an ophthalmologist in the Dutch East Indies. On the other hand during his student years Einthoven had an accident during athletics and broke his wrist, which occasioned his studying of the mechanics of the movements of the elbow. Finally, one of his main investigations as a young professor in physiology concerned the function of the bronchial musculature (as mentioned in chapter 2). All this is true and other research still further away from the cardiac field can be added to this list. To conclude however that therefore Einthoven could equally well have become "an ophthalmologist, orthopaedist or a specialist in respiration disease", and that his final choice for electrocardiography and the invention of the string galvanometer were "fortuitous", is unwarranted if not preposterous. To the great majority of his contemporaries the conclusion was clear. It was the same as adopted here in retrospect: Einthoven had an open mind and many interests. In the beginning he studied several different problems at depth, which he happened to meet; but ultimately

he limited his research largely to electrocardiography and calculated the requirements for the construction of a new galvanometer.

Section 7. The other paper - of much more questionable character because
some of the "facts" given are incorrect or made up - is by James K. Cooper [10]:
"Electrocardiography 100 years ago. Origins, pioneers and contributors." It was
written at the occasion of the centenary of Waller's discovery that the human
cardiac action currents could be led off from the surface of the body. The chief
argument however, concerns Einthoven. While recalling the controversy about
Ader's importance for electrocardiography Cooper quotes Barron: "as these
papers (meaning Ader's only paper as well as those by Rossel subsequently) were
out of Einthoven's field he was unaware of them when he began to develop the
string galvanometer". Nevertheless Cooper concludes: "--- Many people believe
that Einthoven invented the string galvanometer. It is true that he developed
early electrocardiography, but he was not the first to describe the electrocardiogram, and he did not invent the string galvanometer."

The physicist Bosscha is also mentioned as a precursor of Einthoven
because of his construction of a differential galvanometer described in his Latin
thesis of 1854; in addition Cooper calls him Einthoven's teacher and the one who
suggested linking the hospital to the physiological laboratory thereby providing
"both a theoretical and a practical basis for Einthoven's work." The linkage of
laboratory and hospital was discussed in chapter 5 together with information
about Bosscha. Here it should perhaps be recalled, that Bosscha was never a
professor at Leiden; he left that university a few years after his doctoral thesis on
a differential galvanometer (which had nothing to do with Einthoven's concept)
in 1860, the same year that Einthoven was born at Semarang. The reason why
Einthoven started his publication of "Un nouveau galvanomètre" by recalling
Bosscha's thesis was a) that the paper appeared in Bosscha's "Festschrift" (an
issue of the Archives Néerlandaises of which Bosscha was editor) and b) to show
that "Depuis la publication de la thèse de M. Bosscha "De galvanometro differen-
tiali" la technique de la mesure des courants a fait bien de progrès" (This is the
first sentence of Einthoven's paper which can be translated as follows: since the
publication of Mr Bosscha's thesis "About the differential galvanometer" the
technique of measuring currents has made much progress). I must add that
Cooper's paper provoked several letters to the editor in the New England
Journal, but also a paper in the British Heart Journal by Howard Burchell [8],

which provided an excellent answer and is in accordance with the evidence presented here.

Concluding remarks

It is not necessary to make more comments on the different evaluations of Einthoven and his work, apart from emphasizing that there were various factors which contributed to the difference in approach by those who knew Einthoven personally and others who did not; especially if they belonged to a later generation. An important factor was of course oblivion under the dust of time, but later there were also some attempts at a new and provocative approach which occasionally and unfortunately went together with incorrect reading and quoting of Einthoven's writings; moreover, and in this respect several authors are to blame to a varying degree (see chapter 7), with reiterating opinions and pronouncements of others without sufficient checking or critical evaluation.

In fact, my experience with Einthoven's papers and letters has taught me that the only way to properly understand them, is to read them carefully and to take their contents seriously and literally. In particular the latter is important; among other things this means that one must not confuse lack of emphasis with lack of importance nor suspect hidden purposes. It is true (and already mentioned) that Einthoven sometimes omitted to discuss some facts which he considered generally known or self-evident. Also that occasionally he courteously attributed some of his own initiatives to others who were involved in one way or another with their realization (e.g. Bosscha in relation to the electrocardiograms of patients in the hospital; see chapter 5, section 2). In general however, he gave others the (presumably) exact credit that was due to them and, although rarely expressed in so many words, expected the same for himself. Once only he found it necessary to write a short notice of self-defence in Pflüger's Archiv, when he was wrongly accused by Burdon Sanderson of omitting the name of Burch (as mentioned in chapter 2). Perhaps the most important aspect of this episode was not its rarity, but its being short-lived. Although Einthoven initially was really angry and wrote to Julius about it, after the construction of the string galvanometer Burdon Sanderson was very much interested and Einthoven did not mention the old controversy again. In the case of Fahr's paper on the string galvanometer (see chapter 5, section 1) sent up for publication without Einthoven's knowledge, the latter's reaction was still more even handed. It can be noted in this respect that in his correspondence Einthoven seldom and then only mildly defended his priority with respect to the string galvanometer. Even in his letters to Edelmann he did not do so, presumably because he considered Ader's instrument fundamentally different from his own. Probably he was surprised and indignant when the Edelmann's used the resemblance as an excuse to break their contract; in any case he resented that Edelmann Jr took out legal protection for himself on Einthoven's ideas, even if some modification was applied.

The most interesting side of Einthoven's personality in my view is a certain ambiguity: how could this ordinary and conventional man - as Einthoven regarded himself and in some respects certainly was - with traditional (but strong and deep-rooted) virtues like sense of duty, simplicity, and honesty - achieve such extraordinary, far reaching results which are still visible after 100 years? One of the people who found an answer and the fitting words for it, was Fahr [67]: "Einthoven as a man, had an unusual and compelling personality. In a crowd, he was indistinguishable, but, when one saw him in the face, one recognized at once that here was a strong and vital personality - a personality of determination and drive ---".

I refrain from further quotations but perhaps it is interesting to consider what influences from outside favoured Einthoven's work. For one thing, there were some trends in the 19th century, partly going back to the 18th, into which Einthoven's work fitted nicely:

1) replacement or completion of visual observation by graphic and photographic recording,

2) substantiation of causal relations by quantitative observations. In his own case Einthoven stipulated that the electrocardiogram which can be recorded and measured, is well suited to serve as an indication of the function of the unknown biochemical processes which he supposed to be responsible for myocardial contraction.

3) rapid development at the end of the 18th century and throughout the 19th century of electric technology and of electrophysiology from which electro-cardiography formed a link to

4) the gradual but clinically decisive shift from diagnosis post mortem to diagnosis in vivo, initially based on comparing autopsy findings with signs and symptoms of disease, as clearly expressed in the books of Morgagni [93] and Auenbrugger [2] (both published in 1771). Via percussion and Laennec's auscultation this led all the way up to electrocardiography and radiology, which arrived almost simultaneously at the end of the 19th century. It is not necessary to mention that the development did not stop there; the context of this book does not allow further elaboration.

All this may not have been what Einthoven meant, when he said to a friend shortly before his death: "I have always been in luck, both at home and in my work". It is more likely that he thought of Donders, his teacher and model; of Waller who opened the door to the development to electrocardiography but hardly saw the way leading to the future; and of Lewis, who paved that way but got tired of it, perhaps also because he was not sure about the future and may have been disappointed by not sharing the Nobel Prize. It is equally possible, that Einthoven thought of the (then) prevailing university freedom in research, which he praised highly when he wished luck to Julius in a letter of encouragement.

Perhaps Einthoven also was lucky in his genetic inheritance. In the first chapter I referred already to his paternal grandfather and grandmother neither of whom he ever saw: a grandfather with an adventurer's life style by going to war abroad, but who later became a respected surgeon in an era when Dutch surgery shedded its last ties with the barbershop and acquired medical status. At his side a grandmother from an already well established intellectual family, whose father (Willem's great-grandfather) was a physicist and mathematician like his father before him. And nearest to Willem Einthoven: his own father, who showed his love of adventure and of medicine by choosing a medical career in the tropics, but died when Willem was six years old.

Virtually every testimony from Einthoven's friends or acquainted colleagues leads to the conclusion that his achievements were not only due to his intellectual talents (or genius as many said) but also, perhaps foremost, to his strength of character. The latter was specified by de Waart [109] briefly and simply as: "perseverance, modesty, honesty and idealism". Fahr's quotation given above was limited to the first of these qualities, but I think that de Waart was right in his wider choice, as appears also from other testimonies quoted earlier.

I do not want to give the impression that I believe Einthoven was perfect. I hope that my review made clear that some deficiencies, not so much in character as in the deterioration of his initially so exceptional insight and foresight, which particularly with respect to the rapid progress of electrotechnology, began to appear in the last period of his life or even somewhat earlier. These signs were not conspicuous, in fact they probably were invisible to most of his contemporaries because they were masked by the honours and general recognition coming to him in that same period. Of course, increasing age may have started to have its effects.

However, I might add that I sympathize completely with the science reporter, who hoped that the recent accidental discovery of the correspondence between Lorentz and Zeeman (physicist at Amsterdam, joint Nobel prize winner with Lorentz) would reveal some imperfections of the former. So far Lorentz had always been regarded, morally and scientifically, as a model by everybody else, including Einstein as the latter testified himself. But the reporter was disappointed: no indication was found that Lorentz was fallible and therefore human. I must admit my suspicion however, since Lorentz was a pioneer paving part of the way for both Niels Bohr's atomic model and Einstein's theory of relativity, that more diligent search might uncover some evidence of steps which Lorentz could easily have taken, but failed to do. On the other hand Lorentz accepted at the age of 65 years the long (8 years) and difficult task of adviser in the Zuiderzee reclamation scheme. His calculated predictions about the effect on the sea floor at the transition from the unreclaimed part into the North Sea were fully confirmed.

A small but significant indication can be given of Einthoven's "human imperfection". Fahr (l.c.) reports that Einthoven when inspecting an experiment performed by assistants, sometimes took part in a difficult dissection of a nerve. Thereby he wrecked the preparation by tearing the nerve, because he was clumsy with his hands. Fahr may have exaggerated of course, but from conversation with other former assistants I know that there is some truth in Fahr's story. However, they also told me the counterpart of it. When occasionally there was trouble with the string galvanometer which nobody could solve, they would ask Einthoven's advice, even if he was working at home (which he often did for part of the morning). He could nearly always tell how to get the instrument going again without touching or even seeing it. A proof of his practical mind which Samojloff admired together with his theoretical knowledge (chapter 6, section 5) but which did not imply manual dexterity.

Einthoven's personal ideas about the requirements for good research can be deduced from his instruction to new assistants as reported by Hoogerwerf and De Waart (the latter was already quoted on part of this subject). Einthoven asserted that many of those who start scientific work think that they are on the verge of making a series of scientific discoveries. Instead they are going to meet with an endless row of time consuming technical difficulties. As regards himself, he sometimes added that his success was not a result of talent, but of hard work, perseverance and concentration on a limited subject.

Particularly this concentration was essential in Einthoven's view for all average researchers (as Einthoven considered himself and his co-workers). Only a few very exceptionally gifted persons could do excellent work in various fields at the same time, he said, citing Helmholtz and his own teachers Donders and Buys Ballot (the latter was physicist and pioneer meteorologist).

It is interesting to see how in fact Einthoven referred in these words to his own development but overlooked, consciously or not, that he himself had performed the "impossible" prior to 1900 i.e. before his construction of the string galvanometer, which sealed the end of his orientation period.

Einthoven's papers were written and signed by himself. Sometimes the names of assistants were mentioned between brackets: (with ---) or (in collaboration with ---). Occasionally there was noted (after investigations by ---) and once (after joint investigations with ---). In view of other similar events, where Einthoven's reasoning is better known, it seems likely that even in such little details he tried to be as truthful as possible.

Some light on this matter was thrown by Fahr, who recalled that he did some research for Einthoven and wrote a paper about it in 1 month. When he gave it to Einthoven, the latter put it into a drawer, where it remained for a full year. Thereafter it was published after having been rewritten completely by Einthoven.

There is no indication however that Einthoven's assistants felt slighted or neglected. Neither would this have been Einthoven's intention. It has already been mentioned that in his Nobel Lecture Einthoven openly declared his doubt, whether he would have had the privilege of standing there without the valuable contributions of Lewis. He went on by saying: "But in addition, innumerable other workers in the field of electrocardiography have gained great merit. --- A new chapter has been opened in the study of heart diseases, not by the work of a single investigator, but by many talented men, who --- distributed over the whole surface of the earth, have devoted their powers to an ideal purpose, the advance of knowledge, by which, finally, suffering mankind is helped".

References

This list contains the papers by Einthoven which were quoted in this book. For the complete bibliography see no.101.

1. Ader: Sur un nouvel appareil enregistreur pour cables sous-marins. Compt.rend.Acad.Sc. 124: 1440, 1897.

2. Auenbrugger, L.: Inventum Novum, Fascimile edition with translations into French (Corvisaert), English (Forbes) and German (Ungar) and annotations by M.Neuenburger, 1922.

3. Barron, S.L.: The development of the electrocardiograph. Cambridge Monograph No. 5, 1952.

4. Battaerd, P.J.T.A.: Further graphic researches on the acoustic phenomena of the heart in normal and pathological conditions. Heart 6:121, 1915-1917.

5. Bayliss, W.M. & E.H. Starling: On the Electromotive Phenomena of the Mammalian Heart. Int. Monatsch.f.Anat. und Physiol. 9: 256-281, 1892.

6. Biermer, A.: Über bronchial Asthma. Volkmanns Sammlung. Klin. Vorträge,12, 1870.

7. Burch, G.E. & N.P. de Pasquale: A History of Electrocardiography. Chicago, Year Book Medical Publishers, 56-60, 64, 124, 1964.

8. Burchell, H.B.: Did Einthoven invent a string galvanometer? Br. Heart J. 57: 190-193, 1987.

9. Burnett, J.: The origins of the elektrocardiograph as a clinical instrument. Medical History, Supp. no.5: 53-76, 1985.

10. Cooper, J.K.: Electrocardiography 100 years ago: Origins, pioneers and contributors. N. Engl. J. Med. 315:461-464, 1986.

11. Dekker, E., Defares J.G. and Heemstra, H.: The direct measurement of intrabronchial pressure, its application to the location of the check-valve mechanism. J.Appl.Physiol. 13:35, 1958.

12. Dekker, E.: The influence of intrathoracic pressure on the diameter and flow resistance of the airways in normal individuals and in patients with asthma and emphysema. Thesis, 1958.

13. Einthoven, J.F.G.: De Einthoven's wie en wat. 1989. (Privately printed edition).

14. Einthoven, W.: Quelques remarques sur le mécanisme de l'articulation du coude. Arch. néerl. des Sciences Exact. Nat. 17: 289-298, 1882.

15. Einthoven, W.: Stereoscopie door kleurverschil. Proefschrift (Thesis), Utrecht, 4 July 1885.

16. Einthoven, W.: Stéréoscopie dépendant d'une difference de couleur. Arch. néerl. des Sciences Exact. Nat. 20: 361-387, 1886.

17. Einthoven, W.: Der Donders'sche Druck und die Gasspannungen in der Pleurahöhle. Pflügers Arch. ges. Physiol. 44: 152-174, 1888.

18. Einthoven, W.: Het eerste Internationale Physiologen- congres te Bazel (10-12 September 1889). Ned.T.v.Geneesk. 25 II: 457-462; 496-503, 1889.

19. Einthoven, W.: Über die Wirkung der Bronchialmuskeln, nach einer neuen Methode untersucht, und über Asthma nervosum. Pflügers Arch. ges. Physiol. 51: 367- 444, 1892.

20. Einthoven, W.: On the production of shadow and perspective effects by difference of colour. Brain J. Neurol. 16: 191- 202, 1893.

21. Einthoven, W.: Nieuwe methoden voor clinisch onderzoek. Voordracht 44 ste Alg. Verg. der Ned. Maatschappij ter bev. der Geneeskunst [New methods for clinical investigation; paper read at the 4th general meeting of the Dutch medical association]. Ned. T.Geneesk. 29 II: 263-286, 1893.

22. Einthoven, W.: Over Asthma Nervosum. Ned. T.v.Geneesk. II: 469-495, 1893.

23. Einthoven, W. & Geluk M.A.G.: Die Registrierung der Herztöne. Pflügers Arch. ges. Physiol. 57:617, 1894.

24. Einthoven, W.: Über die Form des menschlichen Electrocardiogramms. Pflügers Arch. ges. Physiol. 60: 101-123, 1895.

25. Einthoven, W: Eine Isolationsvorrichtung gegen Erschütterungen der Umgebung. Ann. Physik.Chem. 56: 161- 166, 1895.

26. Einthoven, W.: Vertheidigung gegen J. Burdon Sanderson. Centralbl. Physiol. 9: 277-278, 1895.

27. Einthoven, W.: Physiologie des Rachens. In: Handbuch der Laryngologie und Rhinologie. II Band: Der Rachen, pp.46-64.Wien, Alfred Holder, 1899.

28. Einthoven, W.: Über das normale menschliche Elektrokardiogramm und über die capillär-elektrometrische Untersuchung einiger Herzkranken (mit K. de Lint). Pflügers Arch. ges. Physiol. 80: 139-160, 1900.

29. Einthoven, W.: Un nouveau galvanomètre. Arch. néerl. des Sciences Exact Nat. série 2, 6: 625-633, 1901.

30. Einthoven, W.: Galvanometrische registratie van het menschelijk electro-cardiogram [galvanometric registration of the human electrocardiogram]. In: Herinneringsbundel [remembrance volume] Prof. S.S. Rosenstein, p.101-106. Leiden, Eduard IJdo, 1902.

31. Einthoven, W.: Die galvanometrische Registrierung des menschlichen Elektrokardiogramms, zugleich eine Beurtheilung der Anwendung des Capillär-Elektrometers in der Physiologie. Pflügers Arch. ges. Physiol. 99: 472-480, 1903.

32. Einthoven, W.: In memoriam E.J. Marey. Ned. T .v. Geneesk., 40 I: 109-113, 1904.

33. Einthoven, W.: Le télécardiogramme. Arch.Internat.Physiol. 4:132-164, 1906.

34. Einthoven, W.: The telecardiogram. 1906. Partial translations:
by Mathewson, F.A.L. and Jackh H., Amer.Heart J. 49: 77-82, 1955.
by Blackburn H.W., Amer. Heart J. 53:602-615, 1957.

35. Einthoven, W.: Weiteres über das Elektrokardiogramm. Nach gemeinschaftlich mit Dr. B. Vaandrager angestellten Versuchen mitgeteilt. Pflügers Arch. ges. Physiol. 122: 517-584, 1908.

36. Einthoven, W.: On a third heart sound (in collab with J.H. Wieringa & E.P. Snijders) Proceed. Section Sciences, Kon.Acad.Wet. Amsterdam 10:93-95, 1907/1908.

37. Einthoven, W.: The form and magnitude of the electrical response of the eye to stimulation by light at various intensities (with W.A. Jolly). Quart. J. Exp. Physiol. 1: 373-416, 1908.

38. Einthoven, W.: On vagus currents examined with the string galvanometer (in collab. with A. Flohil and P.J.T.A. Battaerd) Quart. J. Exp. Physiol.1: 243-245, 1908.

39. Einthoven, W.: Über Vagusstrome. Nach gemeinschaftliche mit A. Flohil und P.J.T.A. Battaerd angestellten Versuchen mitgeteilt. Pflügers Arch. ges. Physiol 124: 246-270,1908.

40. Einthoven, W.: Die Konstruktion des Saitengalvanometer. Pflügers Arch. ges. Physiol. 130: 287-321, 1909.

41. Einthoven, W.: Neuere Ergebnisse auf dem Gebiete des tierischen Elektrizität. Verh.Ges.dtsch.Naturf.Aerzte, pp.80-113, 1912.

42. Einthoven, W.: Über die Deutung des Elektrokardiogramms. Pflügers Arch. ges. Physiol.149:65-86, 1912.

43. Einthoven, W.: The different forms of the human electrocardiogram and their signification. (Paper read before the Chelsea Clinical Society on March 19th, 1912). Lancet I: 853-861, 1912.

44. Einthoven, W: On different vagus effects upon the heart investigated by means of electrocardiography (with J.H. Wieringa). Proceed.Section of Sciences, Kon.Acad.Wet. Amsterdam 14: 165-166, 1911/1912.

45. Einthoven, W.: Ungleichartige Vaguswirkungen auf das Herz, elektrokardiographisch untersucht. (mit J.H.Wieringa) Pflügers Arch. ges. Physiol. 149:65-86, 1912.

46. Einthoven, W.: Über die Richtung und die manifeste Grösse der PotentialSchwankungen im menschlichen Herzen und über den Einfluss der Herzlage auf die Form des Elektrokardiogramms (mit G. Fahr und A. De Waart). Pflügers Arch. ges. Physiol. 150:275-315, 1913.

47. Einthoven, W.: On the direction and manifest size of the variations of potential in the human heart and on the influence of the position of the heart on the form of the electrocardiogram (Translated by Hoff H.E. and Sekelj P.) Amer. Heart J, 40:163-211, 1950.

48. Einthoven, W.: On the variability of the size of the pulse in cases of auricular fibrillation (with A.J. Korteweg). Heart 6:107-120, 1915.

49. Einthoven, W.: Über die anglebiche positive Stromschwankung in der Schild-krötenvorkammer bei Vagusreizung nebst Bemerkungen über den Zusammenhang zwischen Kontraktion und Aktionstrom (mit A.C.A. Rademaker). Pflügers Arch. ges. Physiol. 166:109-143, 1916.

50. Einthoven, W.: On the observation and representation of thin threads. Proceed. Section of Science, Kon. Acad. Wet. Amsterdam 23: 705-706, 1920/1921.

51. Einthoven, W.: Über Widerstand und Potentialdifferenz bei dem psycho-galvanischen Reflex (mit J. Roos). Pflügers Arch. ges. Physiol. 189: 126 - 136, 1921.

52. Einthoven, W. Über die Beobachtung und Abbildung dünner Fäden. Pflügers Arch. ges. Physiol.191:60-98, 1921.

53. Einthoven, W.: Über Stromleitung durch den menschlichen Körper (mit J. Bijtel). Pflügers Arch. ges. Physiol. 198: 439-482, 1923.

54. Einthoven, W.: Functions of the cervical sympathetic as manifested by its action currents (with J. Byrne). Amer. J. Physiol. 65: 350-362, 1923.

55. Einthoven, W. & S. Hoogerwerf: Expériences avec le phonographe à corde. Arch. néerl. Physiol. 11: 496-508, 1924.

56. Einthoven, W.: Der Saitenphonograph (mit S. Hoogerwerf), Pflügers Arch. ges. Physiol. 204: 275-294, 1924.

57. Einthoven, W.: The relation of mechanical and electrical phenomena of muscular contraction, with special reference to the cardiac muscle (Lecture Dec. 6 1924) The Harvey Society Lectures 1924-1925 Philadelphia, London, J.B. Lippincott, 1926.

58. Einthoven, W.: La détermination de l'axe électrique du coeur. Acta Paediat. 4:136-140, 1925.

59. Einthoven, W.: Nobel Lecture, December 8, 1925: Das Saitengalvanometer und die Messung der Aktionströme des Herzens.
a. Les Prix Nobel en 1924-1925. Stockholm, P.A. Norstedt & Fils, 1926.
b. Acta Societatis Medicorum Suecanae 51: 213-226, 1926.
c..The string galvanometer and the measurement of the action currents of the heart. Nobel Ed. Physiology or Medicine 1922-1941. Amsterdam, New York, Barking, Elsevier, 1965.

60. Einthoven, W.: Gehirn und Sympathicus VI Mitteilung von Einthoven, Hoogerwerf und Karplus und Kreidl. A. Die Aktionströme des Halssympathicus. Pflügers Arch. ges. Physiol. 215: 443-452, 1927.

61. Einthoven, W.: Die Aktionströme des Herzen (Elektrokardiogramm). In: Handbuch der normalen und pathologischen Physiologie. Ed. A.Bethe et al. pp. 785-862. Berlin, Springer, 1928.

62. Einthoven Jr, W.F.: The string Galvanometer in wireless telegraphy. Pro-ceedings 26. No's 7 and 8, 1923.

63. Einthoven Jr, W.F.: van der Horst, W. en H.Hirschfeld: Brownsche bewe-gingen van een gespannen snaar. Physika 5, 358 - 360, 1925.

64. Erschler, I.: Willem Einthoven - The Man. Arch. Intern Med. 148, Feb 1988.

65. Ewing: Magnetische Induktion. Springer, Berlin 1892.

66. Fahr, G.E.: An analysis of the spread of the excitation wave in the human ventricle . Arch. Int. Med. 25: 146, 1920.

67. Fahr, G.E.: Einthoven. Ik wilde weten.(I wanted to know) Georg Fahr Festschrift. Minneapolis, Lancet Publications, pp. 15-25,1962.

68. Flohil, A.: Proefschrift. Vergelijkende röntgenphoto-graphische en electro-cardiographische onderzoekingen en over de richting en de manifeste grootte van het resulteerend potentiaalverschil in eenige pathologische harten. Drukkerij Pier Westerbaan, Den Haag, 1928.

69. Haas, H.K. de: Thesis. Lichtprikkels en retinastromen in hun quantitatief verband. 1903.

70. Hill, A.V.: Obituary Prof.W.Einthoven. Nature, 120: 591-592, 1927.

71. Hill, A.V.: Trails and trials in physiology. Annual Review of Physiology, 1965.

72. Hollman, A.:. The history of bundle branch block. Medical History, Supp.no.5, 82-102, 1985.

73. Hoogerwerf, S.: W.Einthoven. In Ned. Helden der wetenschap, onder redaktie van T.P. Sevensma, 239, Amsterdam, 1946.

74. Hoogerwerf, S.: W.Einthoven. Dictionary of Scientific Biography. 4, 333-335. Charles Scribner's Sons, New York, 1971.

75. Johansson, J.E.: Nobel Lectures, Physiology or Medicine 1922-1941, including presentation speeches and laureates' biographies. Physiology or Medicine, 1924. Willem Einthoven. Elsevier, Amsterdam 1965:89.

76. Johnston, F.D.& E. Lepeschkin (eds): Selected papers of Dr. F.N. Wilson (Ann Arbor, Mich.Edwards Bros,Inc., 1954).

77. Katz, L. and H.K. Hellerstein: Electrocardiography, in Circulation of the Blood. Men and Ideas. New York, Oxford, (Fishman, A.P. and D.W. Richardson, eds) Chapter V, pp 289-296, 1964.

78. Kekwick, R.A.: Alan Nigel Drury, 3 November 1884 - 2 August 1980. Biographical Memoirs of Fellows of the Royal Society. 27, 173, 1981.

79. Kraus, F., Nicolai, G.F. & F. Meyer: Prinzipielles und Experimentelles über das Elektrokardiogramm. Pflügers Arch. ges. Physiologie. 155: 97 -167, 1914.

80. Krikler, D.M.: Historical Aspects of Electrocardiography. Cardiology Clinics 5 No.3 Aug, 1987.

81. Krikler, D.M.: The search for Samojloff: A Russian physiologist in times of change. Brit. Med. J., 295: 1624-1627,1987.

82. Krikler, D.M.: Alexander Pilipovich Samojloff and Paul Dudley White: Electrocardiography and a Russian-American Friendship. J Am Coll Cardiol, 14:530-531, 1989.

83. Krikler, D.M. and A. Hollman: The last portrait of Willem Einthoven. Newly discovered links between Sir Thomas Lewis and Alexander Samojloff. Br. Heart J. 64: 223-6, 1990.

84. Levine, S.: Willem Einthoven. Some historical notes on the occasion of the centenary celebration of his birth. Am. Heart. J. 6:422-423, 1961.

85. Lewis, T., Meakins, J. and P.D. White: The excitatory process in the dog's heart. Part I. The auricles. Philos. Trans. R. Soc. Ser B 205, 375-420, 1914.

86. Lewis, T. and M.A. Rothschild: The excitatory process in the dog's heart. Part II. The ventricles. Philos. Trans. R. Soc. Ser B 206, 181-226, 1915.

87. Lewis, T: The Mechanism of the Heart Beat (London:Shaw & Sons, 1911).

88. Lewis, T.: Interpretations of the initial phases of the electrocardiogram with special reference to the theory of "limited potential differences" (7th Mellon Lecture),   Arch.Intern Med 30: 269-285, 1922.

89. Lewis, T.: The Mechanism and Graphic Registration of the Heart Beat (3d ed; London: Shaw and Sons) p.104-106, 1925.

90. Lewis, T.: Obituary. Willem Einthoven. Heart, Vol.XIV No.46 Shaw and Sons, London,1927-1929.

91. Mair, A.: Sir James Mackenzie (1853-1925) General Practitioner. Churchill Livingstone, Edinburgh and London,1973.

92. Mann, H.: A method of analyzing the electrocardiogram. Arch. Int. Med. 25:283, 1920.

93. Morgagni J.B.: The seats and causes of diseases investigated by anatomy. Translated from the latin by Alexander B., 1769. Reprinted with introduction by P. Klemperer, 1960.

94. Nolen, W.: Het kenmerkende in het beroep van den geneesheer. Afscheids-college Leiden S.C. van Doesburgh- 1924.

95. Rossel, F.: Télégraphie Sous-Marine. L'éclairage électrique T.XII no.33 pp 295, 1897.

96. Samojloff, A.: Elektrokardiogramme. Sammlung anatomischer und physiologischer Vorträge und Aufsetze. Heft 2. Jena Germany, Verlag von Gustav Fischer, 1-37, 1909.

97. Samojloff, A.: Die positive Schwankung des Ruhestromes am Vorhofe des Schildkrötenherzens bei Vagusreizung (Gaskells Phänomen). Pflügers Arch. ges. Physiol. Bd 199, 1923.

98. Samojloff, A.: Reminiscences of the late Professor Willem Einthoven, Am. Heart. J. 5:545, 1930.

99. Schott, E.: Willem Einthoven und die Fortschritte, welche wir der Erfindung des Saitengalvanometers verdanken. Münchener Med. Wochenschrift. 72 I:391, 1925.

100. Shapiro, E.: Willem Einthoven's Fortuitous Invention. Historical Milestones. Am. J. of Cardiol. 40: 987, 1977.

101. Snellen, H.A.: Selected Papers on electrocardiography of Willem Einthoven. Leiden University Press, 1977.

102. Snellen, H.A.: Two Pioneers of electrocardiography.The correspondence between Einthoven & Lewis 1908-1926. Rotterdam, Donker Academic Publications, 1983.

103. Sykes, A.H.: A.D. Waller and the electrocardiogram. Br.Med.Journal, 294: 1396-1398, 1987.

104. Symes, W.L.: The late Prof. A.D.Waller. Nature, 109:418-419, 1922.

105. Tammeling, G.J.: Willem Einthoven as a pioneer in bronchial function. European Journal of Cardiology, 8/2, 299-302, 1978.

106. Tawara, S.: Das Reizleitungssystem des Säugetierherzens. Ein anatomisch-histologische Studie über das Atrioventricularbundel und die Purkinjeschen Fäden. Jena, Gustav Fischer, 1906.

107. de Vogel, W.Th.: Bijdrage tot de kennis der electrische verschijnselen van het hart. Proefschrift (Thesis), 1893.

108. de Waart, A.: Het levenswerk van Willem Einthoven 1860-1927. Uitgegeven ter gelegenheid van het honderdjarig bestaan der vereniging nederlandsch tijdschrift voor geneeskunde door de erven F.Bohn N.V. Haarlem, 1957.

109. de Waart, A.: Einthoven Commemoration. Am. Heart J. 61:357-360, 1961.

110. Waller, A.D.: A demonstration on man of electromotive changes accom-panying the heart's beat, J.Physiol. 8: 229-234, 1887.

111. Waller, A.D.: On the Electromotive Changes connected with the Beat of the Mammalian Heart in particular. Phil.Trans.Roy.Soc.London. 180:169-194, 1889.

112. Waller, A.D.: Introduction to Human Physiology. London, 1891.

113. Waller, A.D.: The electrocardiogram of man and of the dog as shown by Einthoven's stringgalvanometer. Lancet 1448, 1909.

114. Waller, A.D.: Electrocardiography for clinical purposes. Lancet 379-382, 1913.

115. Waller, A.D.: The Oliver-Sharpey Lectures on the electrical action of the human heart. Lancet pp 21 and 59, 1913.

116. Waller, A.D.: Harvey lecture. New York. Origin and Scope of electrocardio-graphy, 1913.

117. Wenkebach, K.F.: W. Einthoven. D.med.Wschr. 53 II: 2176, 1927.

118. Wiggers, C.J.: Reminiscences and Adventures in Circulation Research. Grune & Stratton, New York & London, 1958.

119. Wiggers, C.J.: Willem Einthoven (1860-1927). Some Facets of His Life and Work. Circ. Res. 9:225-234, 1961.

120. Wilson, F.N.: The distribution of the potential differences produced by the heart beat within the body and at its surface, Am.Heart J. 5: 599, 1930.

121. Wilson, F.N.: MacLeod, A.G. and P.S. Barker: The order of ventricular excitation in human branch block. Am.Heart J. 7:305, 1932.

122. Wilson, F.N.: Published posthumously in Selected Papers. The origin and nature of the progress made in our understanding of the electrocardiogramm during the last three decades. Henri Russel Lecture, 1940.

123. Wilson Lepeschkin, J.: Three cardiologists from a mural. Symposium on Body Surface Mapping of Cardiac Fields, 1972. Adv. Cardiol. Vol.10, pp 11-17 (Karger, Basel 1974).